Medical Histories for the MRCP and Final MB

IQBAL KHAN BSc, PhD, PGCME, MRCP (UK)

Consultant and Honorary Senior Lecturer
Northampton General Hospital

Radcliffe Publishing
Oxford • New York

Radcliffe Publishing Ltd
18 Marcham Road
Abingdon
Oxon OX14 1AA
United Kingdom

www.radcliffe-oxford.com
Electronic catalogue and worldwide online ordering facility.

British Library Cataloguing in Publication Data

A catalogue record for this book is available from the British Library.

ISBN-13: 978 184619 152 7

Typeset by Pindar New Zealand (Egan Reid), Auckland, New Zealand
Printed and bound by Hobbs the Printers Ltd, Southampton, Hampshire, UK

Contents

CONTENTS

*I dedicate this book to Adalat and Maqsuda,
who have worked so very hard over the years.*

Preface

In the modern world we are extremely fortunate in having access to a vast array of technical equipment that enables us to 'probe and prod' people as never before. No doubt this technology is a fantastic asset that lets us treat our patients much more effectively. However, all the equipment in the world is no substitute for a detailed and through medical history, which is key not only to disease diagnosis but also patient management. Hence it is perhaps not surprising that modern medical exams such as the OSCE (Objective Structured Clinical Examination) and the PACES (Practical Assessment of Clinical Examination Skills) for the MRCP (UK) test the ability to take a skilful medical history.

Often candidates feel that taking a medical history is a relatively straightforward task that should not pose any problems, particularly as junior doctors have to routinely take medical histories. However, it isn't as straightforward as often perceived and candidates regularly fail. This is because history taking in real life does not necessarily reflect the artificial scenario of the exam. While on a busy 'medical take' or in a medical clinic running late you usually do not have the time to take a through and rigorous history, which is what is expected in the exam. Moreover, you are not constantly under the gaze of a hawk-eyed examiner (real or imagined). Therefore, work in advance should serve you well. This is particularly true for candidates who have qualified abroad and are not familiar with the medical clerking taught in British medical schools.

Of course, one of the problems facing the candidate is that there is an endless series of potential scenarios that may be encountered. Realistically, it is not possible to go through every conceivable scenario, and to pass the exam it is not necessary to do so. Although mundane, the key to passing is the routine and hence it is crucial that you are totally familiar with all aspects of history taking. You must develop your own personal routine, which needs to be practised again and again. I hope the cases that follow will be helpful in this regard.

While the list of possible scenarios is endless, a few basic rules should help. First and foremost, common things are common and the cases should reflect this. You are much more likely to get a patient with recently diagnosed diabetes mellitus rather than a patient diagnosed with Laurence-Moon-Bardet-Biedl Syndrome. Moreover, the diagnosis is not likely to be anything too acute. For instance, it will be someone with angina rather than someone with an acute myocardial infarct.

You must bear in mind that the examiners are predominantly looking at your history taking skills but in addition you are expected to be familiar with the management of common medical conditions, which should be apparent while you are taking the history. With regards to the MRCP (UK) examination, in the Royal College of Physicians' own words, 'the history taking skills station aims to assess the candidate's ability to gather data from the patient, to assimilate that information and then discuss the case'.

For the exam, most of the time, the case presented will be a new referral. Occasionally it will be someone who is a repeat attendee with possibly a new problem. The skill is to tailor each history to each patient and not act like some automaton. At the end, come up with a summary, differential diagnosis and a further management plan. Bear in mind that the manner in which you take the history may be nearly as important as the actual content. Act compassionately, listen to the patient and pick up verbal and non-verbal cues.

This concise text has been prepared with busy junior doctors and medical students in mind. It is intentionally not long winded and I hope will get you 'up to speed' relatively quickly. I should say that it is not intended as a comprehensive collection of all the possible scenarios that may arise but instead its aim is to introduce you to the sorts of scenarios you are likely to meet in the exam and give you some food for practice. This in turn will hopefully help you pass the exam and go some way towards helping you with your medical careers.

It is strongly recommend that during the weeks and months leading up to the 'big day', you try to spend as much time as possible in role playing with your colleagues, friends or in front of the mirror. Some people find the use of video recording in role play very useful.

At this point I should like to emphasise that all the cases in this book, and the names of doctors, patients and relatives, are fictitious and any similarity to real people and events is by coincidence.

Good luck.

Iqbal Khan
September 2007

Iqbalkhan@doctors.org.uk

About the author

Iqbal Khan is a consultant in gastroenterology and general internal medicine at Northampton General Hospital. He also acts as the Associate Director of undergraduate clinical studies, and is responsible for medical student training within the hospital. He was born in Birmingham and studied at the University of Sheffield. After obtaining a dual honours degree in biochemistry and physiology, he went on to study medicine. He also conducted research with a gastroenterologist for a PhD, and it was this experience that initiated his interest in gastroenterology.

Over the years he has helped many senior house officers to get through their MRCP exams and medical students to get through their finals. He strongly believes that the best way to learn is by teaching others.

Abbreviations

αFP	α-fetoprotein
α1AT	α1-antitrypsin
ACEi	angiotensin-converting enzyme inhibitor
AF	atrial fibrillation
AIDS	acquired immune deficiency syndrome
AMA	anti-mitochondrial antibody
ANA	anti-nuclear antibody
AXR	abdominal X-ray
BCG	bacillus Calmette-Guérin
b.d.	*bis die* (twice daily)
Ca	calcium
CCF	congestive cardiac failure
COPD	chronic obstructive pulmonary disease
CPR	cardiopulmonary resuscitation
CRP	C-reactive protein
CSF	cerebrospinal fluid
CT	computerised tomography
CVA	cerebrovascular accident
CXR	chest X-ray
DH	drug history
DVT	deep vein thrombosis
ECG	electrocardiogram
Echo	echocardiogram
ENT	ear, nose and throat
FBC	full blood count
FH	family history
FVC	forced vital capacity

GGT	gamma-glutamyl transpeptidase
GI	gastrointestinal
GP	general practitioner
Hb	haemoglobin
HIV	human immunodeficiency virus
HPC	history of presenting complaint
IBS	irritable bowel syndrome
IDDM	insulin dependent diabetes mellitus
Ig	immunoglobulin
IM	intramuscular
INR	international normalised ratio
ITU	intensive treatment unit
IV	intravenous
kg	kilogram(s)
LFT	liver function tests
LKM	liver-kidney microsomal
MCV	mean corpuscular volume
mol	mole (quantity of matter)
MRI	magnetic resonance imaging
NSAIDs	non-steroidal anti-inflammatory drugs
o.d./od	*omni die* (once daily)
OGD	oesophagogastroduodenoscopy
PC	presenting complaint
PMH	past medical history
PND	paroxysmal nocturnal dyspnoea
PPI	proton pump inhibitor
prn	*pro re nata*, as required
q.d.s/qds	*quarter die sumendus* (four times daily)
SH	social history
SIADH	syndrome of inappropriate secretion of antidiuretic hormone
SLE	systemic lupus erythematosus
SMA	smooth muscle antibody
TB	tuberculosis
TFT	thyroid function tests
t.i.d./tid	*ter in die* (three times daily)
TTG/tTG	tissue transglutaminase
UE	urea and electrolytes
USS	ultrasound scan
VDRL	venereal diseases research laboratory
WCC	white cell count
Yr(s)	year(s)

How to use this book

This book is designed to provide busy doctors and medical students with common case scenarios, which they can use to practise and develop their history taking skills for the MRCP PACES exam or the medical finals. It is suggested that two or more people work together to practise the cases provided. One of the team can act as the exam candidate and should only be provided with the candidate information, including the GP letter. The other can act as the surrogate patient or relative. It is best to think through the roles and try to make the situation as realistic as possible. Hence they are best practised in a quiet environment.

Work through each case following the format of the exam:

- Spend *two minutes* reading through the case and mentally preparing for the case.
- The discussion should take *14 minutes*.
- Allow *one minute* for reflection.
- The examiners have *five minutes* to question you on the case.
- Total time for each case is 22 minutes (*20 minutes* in the exam room).

Once a case has been conducted, the discussion can be reviewed. There are infinite permutations that any 14-minute medical discussion can follow which depend upon a number of variables. These include the medical facts available and the individual's communication and linguistic skills. Medical exams such as the MRCP and the final MB follow formats where pattern recognition is the key to success. Practise and you will succeed.

PART 1

Taking a Medical History

THE OBJECTIVES

The key objectives of a medical history include:
- establishing a rapport with the patient
- clarifying the nature of the patient's ailment and their perception of the illness
- identifying possible organs or systems involved and to then focus the clinical examination
- comprehending the social context of the illness. Namely what impact the illness has on the patient's life and the impact of 'life' on the patient's symptoms
- identifying the patients expectations.

To achieve these objectives the doctor needs to be able to take a detailed and effective medical history within a limited amount of time. It is essential to realise the significance of time and its importance in determining whether or not you will pass or fail the exam. Any competent layperson should be able to take a comprehensive medical history if given enough time and a performa outlining the questions to ask. However, during busy clinics and acute medical takes, the skilful doctor should be able to carry out the same task over a few minutes and formulate a plan of action. This skill is developed by practising and fine tuning your technique so that irrespective of the case you are presented with at the exam, you can take a detailed medical history, outline an action plan and present it to the examiners – all in the space of about 20 minutes.

Inspection of the MRCP PACES mark sheet (readily accessible on the MRCP (UK) website at http://www.mrcpuk.org/Examiners/Documents/Station_2.pdf) for the history taking station shows that the candidates will essentially be examined in three areas:
1 data gathering in the interview
2 identification and use of the information gathered
3 discussion related to the case.

These will now be discussed in greater detail. Final MB examiners will use similar mark sheets and hence medical students may also choose to use these sheets while practising their skills.

1. DATA GATHERING IN THE INTERVIEW

The examiners will expect you to perform the following tasks.

- Elicit the presenting complaint and document all associated symptoms logically and systematically. Find out about any relevant psychosocial factors. For instance, it is very relevant if a patient presents with headaches and you find out that these symptoms started shortly after she found out that her husband was having an affair!
- Take a detailed past medical, drug, social and family history.
- Display appropriate verbal and non-verbal communication with a good balance of open and closed questions and behave in an appropriate manner.

It is essential to note that the history needs to be taken in a logical and systematic manner. Over the course of your training most of you will have developed a system for taking a medical history. And if you are happy with the format, please stick with it as long as you incorporate the above tasks. For those of you that are not happy with your history taking skills or are in the process of developing your skills, I present a possible scheme here:

Taking a medical history
Presenting complaint (PC)
State the problem that has prompted the medical referral, e.g. shortness of breath, chest pain, double vision etc.

History of the presenting complaint (HPC)
Elaborate on the presenting complaint. This is the most important part of the history and should yield the most relevant information and hence appropriately more time should be allotted to this portion of the history. The doctor has to encourage the patient to start talking about their medical problems by asking *open questions* or statements such as 'Your doctor has referred you here because of your medical problems, tell me more', 'What is your medical problem?' A common error is to ask too many questions and thus afford the patient little opportunity to give the history. So, *let the patient talk*. However, time is precious so it is important that the patient doesn't waste time by talking about issues that are not relevant to the presenting complaint. Patients have to be 'kept on

track' with suitable interjections. In any case the occasional remark such as 'Tell me more' and 'Go on' will aid in eliciting a history, particularly when the patient is reticent. As the consultation continues, more specific and *closed questioning* will become necessary to elicit a more detailed history: 'Does the pain go down your arms or up into your neck?', 'What caused you to develop the breathing difficulties?', 'Was the pain sharp or dull in nature?' An important point to bear in mind is that questions should not be leading.

Past medical history (PMH)

Enquire about other illnesses that the patient is suffering with or has suffered with in the past. Also enquire about any previous operations that the patient may have had. You can develop a 'sieve' of common conditions that can be specifically enquired about; for instance, hypertension, asthma, epilepsy, diabetes, angina, peptic ulcer disease etc. Try not to rush through a list as you will leave the patient confused and the examiners will not be too impressed. Remember also that much of this ground will be covered in the systems enquiry below.

Drug history (DH)

Although many people will suggest that you proceed to a systemic/ systems enquiry at this stage, I feel that it is more logical instead to ask about the patient's current medications, including the dosing. Also ask about any known drug allergies and use this opportunity to enquire about allergies to other substances. It is also essential that you remember to ask about over-the-counter medicines.

Social and personal history (SH)

This is an opportunity to really get to know the patient. Ensure that you have enquired about the patient's occupation and, if appropriate, any bearing it may have on their illness. For instance, if someone has presented with abnormal liver biochemistry and it transpires that they work as a pub landlord, it would perhaps be logical to ask whether this results in them consuming excessive amounts of alcohol. Generally, in any patient it is important that you specifically ask about cigarette smoking and alcohol consumption. It is also worth enquiring into the patient's social set up, i.e. who they live with and in what sort of house. In the UK, there is a major problem with delayed discharge of elderly patients for social reasons once they are deemed medically fit for discharge. Hence, it is particularly important to take a detailed social history in elderly patients. Examiners will be very impressed if you do. Particularly ask about their activities of daily living (ADL) such as cooking, washing and shopping, whether they do this themselves or receive help from family/friends or social services. In some instances (for example, where sexually transmitted diseases or blood borne viral illness is suspected) it may be appropriate to take a sexual history and ask about illicit drug use. But it should not be part of the routine history. It is important to tease out the relevant information without appearing to be prying. This is particularly true if a sexual history, such as the number of partners, episodes of unprotected sex and sexual orientation, needs to be taken. With certain conditions, particularly infectious diseases, a travel history should also be elicited.

Family history (FH)

It is important to ask about illnesses that run in the family. For example a young patient may present with a diarrhoeal illness and it is crucial that you ask about other family members suffering with inflammatory bowel disease. It is worth asking about the circumstances of the deaths of first-degree relatives such as parents and siblings. Where an inherited illness is suspected, consider constructing a genetic tree illustrating the involvement of various family members.

Systems enquiry/review (SE)

Now you can ask about each system in turn, and ensure that there is no important information that has been omitted.

- *Cardiovascular:* chest pain, palpitations, pedal oedema, nocturnal dyspnoea?
- *Respiratory:* shortness of breath, haemoptysis, cough, sputum?
- *Gastrointestinal:* appetite, weight loss, abdominal pain, altered bowel habit?
- *Neurology:* headaches, speech, visual or gait problems?
- *Genito-urinary:* dysuria, nocturia, frequency, discharge, menstrual problems?

Communication skills

The interview should be entirely *purposeful*. The questions should not be simply conversational or leading, but should be probing and relevant. It is important that you listen to the patient and at least seem to be very attentive. Rapport is better and patients are more forthcoming with information if they feel that the doctor is listening. Good listening aids empathy (putting yourself in the patient's shoes). *Active listening* is demonstrated by the use of eye contact, posturing (e.g. head nodding) and responding or asking, directly after the patient's last response.

For the interview to be purposeful, it is important that you encourage the patient to remain relevant to the purpose of the interview and redirect them if they go off at a tangent. If there is any doubt about a response it is OK to ask the patient for clarification. Sometimes, patients find it difficult to articulate their true problems and concerns, and both verbal and nonverbal cues help to shed more light on the underlying problem. An example of a *verbal cue* may be a patient who has presented with heartburn and during the course of the consultation may say, 'My mother suffered with heartburn and turned out to have stomach cancer.' This patient may not be particularly bothered about the heartburn and instead be seeking reassurance that he does not have cancer. The good doctor can glean much information from a patient's gait, posture and general body language – so-called *nonverbal* cues. For example, excessive eye contact may suggest anger and aggression, whereas lack of eye contact can imply embarrassment and depression.

Appropriate *touch* (handshake, putting arm around a distressed person) is also a powerful means of communication, building rapport and showing empathy. No doubt some people find it easier to use touch than others. As a general rule, avoid excessive touching, particularly if you are someone who is not comfortable with touching other people.

2. IDENTIFICATION AND USE OF INFORMATION GATHERED

Normally after the medical history is taken you start to examine the patient. However, in this artificial set up of the PACES exam or an OSCE, you have to conclude proceedings at this juncture. If there is any uncertainty, check that the information is correct with the patient and proceed to summarise the history and produce a list of likely differential diagnoses; formulate a management plan and any investigations that may be necessary. It is always nice to ask the patient if they have any questions. The examiners will be particularly keen to see that you have produced a list of the main problems and your ability to correctly interpret the history.

3. DISCUSSION RELATED TO THE CASE

In a nutshell, the examiners will be assessing your ability to discuss the implications of the patient's problems and your strategy for solving these problems.

PART 2

Practice Cases

CASE 1: SUDDEN BLINDNESS

Candidate information

You are reviewing patients in the medical outpatient clinic. Your next patient has been referred by his general practitioner with the following letter. Please read the letter and then review the patient.

Dear Doctor,

Re: Ronald Smith

Thank you for seeing this 48-year-old gentleman. He recently experienced painless loss of sight in his right eye for approximately 10 minutes. The sight recovered spontaneously and he has not had any further problems since then.

I have been treating him for hypertension with atenolol 100 mg od, but this remains poorly controlled. He is a smoker of 30 cigarettes/day and I suspect he has a heavy alcohol intake. Please advise on the further management for this man.

Many thanks for your advice.

Yours sincerely,

Subject/Patient's information

Name: Mr Ronald Smith
Age: 48 years
Occupation: Unemployed

Three weeks ago, while making a cup of tea this man noticed sudden loss of sight in his right eye. There was no associated pain and it was like a cloud had come over his vision. There was no problem with the other eye or any other part of his body. During the episode, he felt a little dizzy and panicked and went into the living room and sat down. After 10 minutes or so the vision returned to normal. This problem had never occurred previously or since then.

His past medical history includes a diagnosis of hypertension after he went to see his GP with headaches, some years ago. Blood tests carried out last year had shown cholesterol of 6.2 mmol/L and his GP had advised Mr Smith to cut down his fat intake (he is very fond of fried food). His appendix was removed as a child.

He has a prescription of atenolol 100 mg once daily, but frequently forgets to take them. There are no known allergies to any drugs.

He started smoking at the age of 13 years and now smokes 30–40 cigarettes a day. Lives alone and is unemployed. His last job was 14 years ago in a bakery. He tends to socialise in the local pub on a daily basis and tends to drink 4–5 pints of beer each evening. His father died of a heart attack at the age of 52 years but the mother is 72 years old and well, apart from troublesome osteoarthritis. There is little contact with his two brothers, who as far as he knows are well.

Data gathering in the interview
- Greet the patient and introduce yourself.
- Confirm that the patient was referred by his GP because of loss of vision and go into the details. Particularly ask about the nature of the blindness: whether it was partial or complete? Was it sudden or more like a 'curtain being drawn over the visual field'? Was there any pain or an associated headache? Have there been any previous or subsequent episodes?
- Ask about the past medical history. Confirm the history of hypertension and ask about any previous history of diabetes mellitus, atrial fibrillation, coagulopathies (such as polycythaemia) and diagnosis of hypercholesterolaemia.
- Drug history and allergies. Is he on aspirin or warfarin?
- Take the social history: Confirm the smoking habit and go into details of the alcohol consumption. In this instance it is important to ask about any previous history of intravenous drug abuse. Ask about his employment.
- Ask about any history of illness in the family. In Afro-Caribbean patients you should ask about any history of sickle cell disease.
- Make the systems enquiry.
- Now confirm that the information is correct and create a problem list and a possible management plan.

Discussion related to the case
This gentleman suffered a transient loss of vision. The most likely causes

for this are either a transient ischaemic episode or amaurosis fugax. Other possibilities include migraine or a vasculitis, such as giant cell arteritis, but these are unlikely in this instance as there was no associated pain.

Both transient ischaemic episodes and amaurosis fugax can be due to embolic, thrombotic, vasospastic, or haematological phenomena. The first two are the most likely contenders for this man. Typically, the visual loss is painless and lasts for 2–30 minutes and resolves completely.

The examiners will be interested in your strategy for managing this patient. The following is a suggested plan.

- Examination of the patient. This should include fundoscopy, listening for carotid bruits and heart murmurs. In addition, blood pressure should be checked and urine dipstick performed to check for diabetes.
- Blood tests:
  - full blood count – to check for polycythaemia and thrombocytosis
  - serum lipids
  - fasting glucose and consider an oral glucose tolerance test
  - inflammatory markers, particularly ESR.
- CT or MRI of the head.
- Carotid dopplers and an echocardiogram.

Management will depend on the findings of the investigations. For instance, if carotid stenosis is proven, the patient will benefit from a carotid endarterectomy. Anti-platelet agents (e.g. aspirin, clopidogrel) and lipid lowering therapies have proven benefit in transient ischaemic episodes. It is also worth pointing out that the specialist skills of ophthalmologists and stroke specialists may be required.

CASE 2: PAINFUL KNEE

Candidate information

You are reviewing patients in the medical outpatient clinic. Your next patient has been referred by his general practitioner with the following letter. Please read the letter and then review the patient.

Dear Doctor,

Re: Jason Gammet

I would be grateful for your advice regarding this 27-year-old chap who works as a mechanic. He is complaining of sore eyes and severe pain in his left knee, which is affecting his work. On examination I find that he does indeed have red eyes and his left knee is swollen. I have requested an X-ray and have suggested that he takes regular paracetamol for now.
   Many thanks for your expert advice.

Yours sincerely,

Subject/Patient's information

Name: Mr Jason Gammet
Age: 27 years
Occupation: Mechanic

Over the past couple of weeks this man has noticed a very uncomfortable gritty sensation in his eyes and progressive swelling and pain in his left knee. There are no other joints affected, although he has noticed mild back pain. He is still able to continue with his work as a mechanic, although there is difficulty in kneeling. Of greater concern to him is the pain that he feels on urination and has noticed a penile discharge and a rash on the glans of the penis (this information should only be volunteered if specifically asked for by the doctor). Because of these symptoms he is concerned that he may have a sexually transmitted disease (and possibly AIDS) and indeed he did have unprotected sex three weeks previously after meeting a woman in a nightclub.

He is not in a steady relationship, but has had several short-term or casual relationships over the years. He has not noticed any change in bowel habit. However, he does tend to suffer with intermittent episodes of diarrhoea and bloatedness associated with lower abdominal pain and cramps.

The past medical history is otherwise unremarkable and he has never been admitted to hospital. He is not taking any medication regularly. There are no known allergies. He smokes cigarettes occasionally and tends to drink about 30 units of alcohol each week. He lives with his parents who are both fit and well, although his mother has previously been diagnosed with celiac disease and is being followed up as an outpatient.

Data gathering in the interview

- Greet the patient and introduce yourself.
- Invite him to tell you about his medical problems and the reason for his referral. Ask details about his specific ailments such as the sore eyes and knee pain. The combination of arthritis and conjunctivitis should alert you to the possibility of a seronegative arthropathy such as Reiter's syndrome at an early stage and hence you should specifically enquire about bowel and genitourinary symptoms. At this stage it may be appropriate to follow the patient's lead and tactfully take a sexual history, which would be appropriate in the context of the possible underlying diagnosis. You may even use this as ploy to acquire the sexual history. For example, *'Symptoms of the sort you describe can sometimes be due to sexually transmitted infections. Can you tell me whether you are in a steady relationship?'*
- Past medical history. Is there a history of spondyloarthritides/HLA-B27 associated disorders, e.g. ankylosing spondylitis, inflammatory bowel disease, psoriatic arthritis.
- Drug history and allergies. Specifically ask about any over-the-counter medicines that the patient may have tried for his symptoms and whether these have proved useful.
- Take the social history. Ask about his employment and what impact his symptoms are having on his work.
- Ask about any history of illness in the family. Particularly ask about history of illnesses associated with HLA-B27, such as ankylosing spondylitis, psoriatic arthropathy, inflammatory bowel disease etc.
- Make the systems enquiry.

- Now confirm that the information is correct and create a problem list and a possible management plan.

Discussion related to the case

This case illustrates a number of areas where the candidate should be competent in eliciting a detailed history. These include the sexual and the locomotor histories.

The sexual history

There is often a great deal of embarrassment and anxiety for patients when giving details of their sexual practices. The situation will only be exacerbated by a doctor who is uncomfortable in taking a sexual history. When taking a sexual history, thinks of the *p's*:

- Preference. Is the patient heterosexual, homosexual or bisexual?
- Protection. Do they tend to use condoms?
- Practice. Are they in a steady relationship, have several partners or practise casual sex?
- Problems. Have they noticed any symptoms that may be of concern, e.g. discharge, rash, dysuria etc?

The locomotor history

When taking a locomotor/rheumatological history it is important not only to get an idea of the severity of symptoms, but also the degree of disability caused by these. The doctor taking the history should assess whether a single joint (monoarthritis) or several joints (polyarthritis) are involved. Along the same lines, get an idea of whether the disease is symmetrical or asymmetrical. Does it affect the large joints, small joints or both, and is it inflammatory or non-inflammatory? Enquire specifically about the following symptoms.

- **Pain:** This is the commonest reason that patients seek medical advice. The severity of pain may not be related to the degree of deformity or disability. As a general rule, pain due to inflammation gets better with activity and hence usually the symptoms improve during the course of the day. On the other hand, pain due to degenerative changes worsens during the course of the day. Rheumatological pain is usually associated with movement and is often referred. For example, a patient with a degenerative hip may present with a painful knee.
- **Swelling:** Inflammatory conditions such as rheumatoid arthritis are associated with *synovial swelling*, which is soft and boggy and is hot

and tender to touch. Degenerative conditions such as osteoarthritis cause *bony swelling* with no obvious associated heat and the swelling is not obviously tender to touch. *Fluctuant swelling* is due to the presence of fluid in the joint.

- **Stiffness:** Rheumatological conditions lead to stiffness in the joint where the patient finds it difficult to mobilise the joint after a period of rest. For obvious reasons, the problem tends to be worst first thing in the morning.
- **Deformity:** This is best judged by inspection at the time of examination and implies long-standing arthritis.
- **Disability:** This is very subjective for the patient and doctors (including MRCP candidates.) will be caught out by assuming severe disability simply because there is deformity. Patients generally adapt to long-standing illness and may be able to carry out complex tasks. A consultant once told me that he was amazed to find out that a patient that was referred to him with advanced rheumatoid arthritis continued to work as a lift engineer, which frequently involved him climbing up the lift shaft using the cable.
- **Systemic illness:** This includes symptoms of fever, weight loss, lethargy and rashes.

The distribution of the arthritis and the associated symptoms will help to establish a likely clinical diagnosis.

Reiter's syndrome

This condition usually affects young men, where the HLA-B27 genotype is a predisposing factor. The resultant reactive polyarthritis frequently follows a genitourinary infection with *Chlamydia trachomatis*, or less frequently enteric infections (e.g. some strains of salmonella and shigella). Clinical features consist of a triad of a seronegative arthritis, conjunctivitis and urethritis. Low back pain secondary to a reactive sacroiliitis is common. Other features include oral ulceration, circinate balanitis, plantar fascitis, iritis, keratoderma blennorrhagica and rarely aortic incompetence. Diagnosis is clinical and blood tests may show non-specific abnormalities such as a normocytic anaemia and raised inflammatory markers. Synovial fluid examination shows a neutrophilia. X-ray examination is generally normal, except in chronic disease, when degenerative changes may be present. Management is with rest and NSAIDs. Occasionally, intra-articular steroid injections may be useful. Antibiotics (e.g. doxycycline) may shorten the course of the condition when it is due to chlamydia. The disease has a variable course, but recovery usually takes months and some patients may remain symptomatic for years.

Other differential diagnoses to consider in this man include: gonococcal arthritis, gouty arthritis, Still's disease, rheumatic fever, psoriatic arthritis and rheumatoid arthritis.

CASE 3: DIARRHOEAL ILLNESS

Candidate information

You are reviewing patients in the medical outpatient clinic. Your next patient has been referred by her general practitioner with the following letter. Please read the letter and then review the patient.

Dear Doctor,

Re: Ms Lucy Fenwick

Age: 25 years

Thank you for seeing the young PhD student who has been suffering with diarrhoea since her return from India three months ago. There is little weight loss but her appetite is not as good as usual. I carried out some blood tests and will forward the results to you when available. Stool cultures have been sent but leaked in transit to the labs. Please advise if she needs a sigmoidoscopy.

Yours sincerely

Subject/Patient's information

Name: Lucy Fenwick
Age: 25 years
Occupation: PhD student

This lady has suffered with diarrhoea for approximately three months. It started four weeks after her return from a month long holiday in India. Normally she opens her bowels 1–2 times a day but over this period of time it has increased to 6–10 times a day. On a few occasions there has been a small amount of fresh blood, mixed with the stools. Also present is mild abdominal pain associated with bloating and cramps. Appetite has not been as good as usual and she has noticed a 10 lb weight loss.

In the past she has enjoyed good health and has never been admitted to hospital. She takes no prescribed medication but is in the habit of taking one multivitamin capsule each evening (bought over the counter). However, a few weeks before the diarrhoea started, she had developed a sore throat and her GP had prescribed a short course of antibiotics. There are no known allergies. She has never smoked and drinks approximately six glasses of red wine per week.

Family history of illness includes an aunt with celiac disease and a cousin with colitis (the details are not known but the cousin had undergone a major bowel operation). Both parents are alive and well. She split with her long term boyfriend two years previously and has not had a relationship since this time and lives alone.

Miss Fenwick is very worried that there may be something serious going on, including the possibility of cancer. She is also worried about the impact of this illness on her studies.

Data gathering in the interview

- Greet the patient and introduce yourself.
- Tell the patient that you have received a letter from her GP regarding her diarrhoea and invite her to tell you more about this. Ensure that you have details on the frequency and nature (formed, watery, steatorrhoea) of the diarrhoea and get details of any bleeding. Is the blood bright red/fresh or altered/old blood? Is it only seen when she wipes herself? Also ask about any weight loss and changes in appetite (always confirm the information on the GP letter).
- Take past medical history.
- Drug history and allergies. Specifically ask about any antibiotics that she may have taken. Is she taking any medication (e.g. loperamide) to control the diarrhoea?
- Take the social history. Has there been any foreign travel? Are there any contacts who have diarrhoea?
- Ask about any history of illness in the family. Specifically ask about gastrointestinal illness. Young patients may have parents who died young of bowel cancer leading to the possibility of inherited illness such as familial adenomatous polyposis coli. But, more significantly, a family history of inflammatory bowel disease has to be sought.
- Make the systems enquiry.
- Now confirm that the information is correct and create a problem list and a possible management plan.

Discussion related to the case

There are many causes of diarrhoea in this lady, but a careful clinical history would serve well to elucidate the likely aetiology. The possibilities to consider include the following.

- **Functional diarrhoea.** Irritable bowel syndrome is very common in young women and can be precipitated by infection. Patients usually complain of lower abdominal pain, bloating, urgency, a feeling of incomplete evacuation and a change in bowel habit. This can be either diarrhoea or constipation. Patients with irritable bowel syndrome usually put weight on, which is not the case here. But IBS cannot be excluded on the basis of weight loss, particularly as the rectal bleeding noted could simply be due to perianal disease such as piles.

- **Inflammatory bowel disease.** Ulcerative colitis and Crohn's disease should always be considered in a young person presenting with new diarrhoea, particularly if it is a bloody diarrhoea. Moreover, this lady has a family history of inflammatory bowel disease, albeit in a second degree relative.

- **Infective causes.** Bacterial (e.g. salmonella, shigella, campylobacter) and viral (e.g. rotavirus, astrovirus, Norwalk-like viruses) infections can lead to diarrhoeal illness. But the incubation period is generally a few days and is not likely to have caused the illness in this woman. *Giardia lamblia* is a flagellate protozoan, which lives in the duodenum and jejunum and is transmitted via the faeces. It tends to be acquired by drinking contaminated water and is a likely culprit for diarrhoea in a traveller returning from India. However, the incubation period is relatively short (1–2 weeks) and patients tend to complain of upper gut symptoms such as bloating, nausea and early satiety. Amoebiasis (due to *Entamoeba histolytica*) can have an extremely long incubation period, but produces an illness with profuse and bloody diarrhoea. It is noteworthy that this lady took a course of antibiotics before the diarrhoea started. This makes pseudomembranous colitis caused by overgrowth of *Clostridium difficile* a potential cause for her symptoms.

- **Small bowel disease.** Enteropathies such as gluten sensitive enteropathy (celiac disease) and tropical sprue should be considered. Simple bacterial overgrowth is a less likely proposition, as this tends to affect vulnerable patients such as neonates, elderly and those with previous upper GI surgery or anatomic anomaly.

- **Pancreatic insufficiency.** This would cause a steatorrhoea, which is not the case here.
- **Non-GI cause.** Always think 'outside the box' and there are many non-GI causes of diarrhoea in a young woman. These include thyrotoxicosis, drugs (laxative abuse, alcohol, digoxin etc), fictional/psychogenic and autonomic neuropathy (unlikely in this case).

Investigations

The investigations for any diarrhoeal illness should be guided by the clinical history and examination. Useful investigations for this woman include the following.

- Blood tests:
  - FBC: the white cell count may be elevated in infective diarrhoea. Bleeding or enteropathy may cause anaemia and in inflammatory illnesses the platelets may be elevated
  - Inflammatory markers: ESR and CRP will be elevated in inflammatory illness
  - Urea and electrolytes to check to see if the patient is dehydrated
  - Albumin will be reduced in any severe illness or if there is a protein losing enteropathy
  - Endomysial and TTG antibodies to look for celiac disease.
- Stool cultures: Multiple sets should be sent for microscopy, culture and sensitivity analysis and the lab should be specifically instructed to look for ova, cysts, parasites and *Clostridium difficile* toxins.
- It is perhaps mandatory to proceed to a rigid or flexible **sigmoidoscopy** in this patient to look for evidence of an active colitis and to take biopsies.

If these tests fail to reveal the cause of this patient's symptoms, further tests may become necessary. These could include gastroscopy (to take duodenal aspirates and biopsies) and small bowel barium studies (to look for anatomical anomalies such as diverticuli or structuring)

Management

Management would depend upon the underlying cause.

CASE 4: HAEMOPTYSIS

Candidate information
You are reviewing patients in the medical outpatient clinic. Your next patient has been referred by his general practitioner with the following letter. Please read the letter and then review the patient.

Dear Doctor,

Re: Mr Ibrar Siddique

Age: 42 years

I am very concerned about this Asian gentleman who presented complaining of a long-standing cough and has recently noticed haemoptysis. I am worried that there is sinister underlying pathology. Because of the urgency of this referral I have been unable to organise a chest X-ray. But I would, nonetheless, very much like your advice on the further investigation and management of this chap.

Yours sincerely

Subject/Patient's information
Name: Mr Ibrar Siddique
Age: 42 years
Occupation: Waiter

This gentleman has been a smoker since the age of 17 years. Over the last few years, he has noticed a cough particularly in the morning, which he has attributed to his smoking habit. Unfortunately, over the past few months the cough has worsened. It is a dry cough but on two occasions he has noticed fresh and altered blood in his sputum, in the morning. Over this period of time he has also felt lethargic and run down. On numerous occasions, during the night, he has had to get out of bed to change his clothing, which had become drenched in sweat. Colleagues and family have commented on weight loss. The gentleman doesn't weigh himself but has noted that he tends to wear his belt two notches up from his previous normal position.

At the age of 15 years he suffered with malaria while living in Pakistan. He immigrated to the UK at the age of 17 years, and since then has been fit and well. He does not take any medications and is not known to be allergic to any medicines. If questioned, he does not recall ever been immunised against TB, and has no scar on his arm.

He does not consume alcohol or use any illicit drugs. He lives with his wife and four children, the youngest of which is eight months old. There is no family history of illness. Mother is alive and well, currently living in Pakistan but father died when he was a baby, following an industrial accident. Mr Siddique has not travelled abroad since his arrival to the UK and has no contacts who have TB.

He is very worried that he may be suffering with lung cancer. TB is less of a worry as he regards this as an easily treatable condition. But he is worried that he may end up losing his job and consequently has not mentioned his symptoms to his work colleagues.

Data gathering in the interview
- Greet the patient and introduce yourself.
- Invite him to tell you about his medical problems and the reason for his referral. Ask about the duration of the cough and haemoptysis. Ask about the nature of the haemoptysis: Is it fresh or altered blood? And get an idea of the quantity. Ask about the weight loss and ask the patient to quantify it. Ask about other systemic symptoms such as lethargy, fever and night sweats.
- Past medical history. Ask about any history of tuberculosis and history of previous BCG vaccination. Has he previously had a chest X-ray showing any abnormality?
- Drug history and allergies.
- Take the social history. Go into details of the smoking history and try to quantify the pack years.
- Ask about any history of illness in the family. Again specifically ask about contacts and family members who may have suffered with tuberculosis.
- Make the systems enquiry. Look for genitourinary, gastrointestinal and neurological symptoms that may be attributable to TB. Remember, it is not just a respiratory condition.

● Now confirm that the information is correct and create a problem list and a possible management plan.

Discussion related to the case

In summary this is a 42-year-old Asian man who is a smoker and has developed haemoptysis, weight loss, lethargy and night sweats. The main differential diagnosis here lies between pulmonary TB and lung cancer. The first line investigations should include random sputum smears to look for alcohol and acid fast bacilli and a chest X-ray. Treatment may be initiated on the basis of these and a typical clinical history. However, for more definitive tests we require a positive sputum culture.

If doubts remain about the diagnosis after preliminary investigations (which should include blood tests such as clotting and a full blood count), it would be pertinent for a chest physician to consider a bronchoscopy or organise more detailed radiological imaging.

CASE 5: NEW DIABETIC

Candidate information

You are reviewing patients in the medical outpatient clinic. Your next patient has been referred by her general practitioner with the following letter. Please read the letter and then review the patient.

Dear Doctor,

Re: Mrs Elizabeth Chapman

Age: 46 years

Please review and advise on the management of this lady who has been complaining of polydipsia and weight loss. A random finger prick glucose carried out by our practice nurse was 11.4.

Yours sincerely

Subject/Patient's information

Name: Mrs Elizabeth Chapman
Age: 46 years
Occupation: School dinner lady

This lady has been suffering with lethargy for some months, which seems to be progressively worsening. In addition, she has also noticed symptoms of severe thirst, frequent urination (including several times during the night) and blurred vision on a few occasions.

Her doctor is currently treating her for hypertension with a beta-blocker. The hypertension is likely to be related to her obesity, which isn't helped by her vocation as she tends to nibble throughout the day, while working as a school dinner lady. She has suffered with depression in the past, following a divorce, and is also taking amitriptyline. She is not on any other medication and has no known allergies. She drinks approximately 20 units of alcohol each week and smokes 10 cigarettes per day. There is no history of illness in the family. There are no children and she lives alone.

Data gathering in the interview

- Greet the patient and introduce yourself.
- Invite the patient to tell you about her medical problems and the reason for his referral. Ask in depth about specific symptoms such as polydipsia, polyuria, lethargy and blurred vision. Try to quantify the weight loss.
- Past medical history. Is the hypertension well controlled? Are there any other 'macro-vascular' risk factors such as smoking, hypercholesterolaemia, family history.* Has she any history of renal impairment?
- Drug history and allergies.
- Take the social history. Go into details of the smoking history and try to quantify the pack years.
- Ask about any history of illness in the family. Does anybody in the family suffer with diabetes?
- Make the systems enquiry.
- Now confirm that the information is correct and create a problem list and a possible management plan.

Discussion related to the case

This is a relatively straightforward history scenario and most candidates would relish the prospect of such a case. The problem is, however, that the examiners will expect greater awareness and knowledge of common conditions such as diabetes mellitus and will therefore expect the data gathering and interpretation to be comprehensive.

---

* It is important that you are not too rigid with the sequence in which the history is taken. Sometimes it is logical to combine different areas of the medical history. For instance, in this case we can take the smoking history, family history and past medical history together in an attempt to quantify the patient's risk of developing macrovascular complications (stroke, ischaemic heart disease etc).

CASE 6: SHORTNESS OF BREATH

Candidate information

You are reviewing patients in the medical outpatient clinic. Your next patient has been referred by his general practitioner with the following letter. Please read the letter and then review the patient.

Dear Doctor,

Re: Mr Kenneth McDonald

Age: 56 years

This man has been complaining of shortness of breath for the last three months. It seems to be getting worse. He also suffers with hypertension, but this seems to be well controlled at present. A chest X-ray I requested appears to be unremarkable, but I am awaiting a formal report. Please advise if he needs further investigation or treatment. Many thanks for your assistance.

Yours sincerely

Subject/Patient's information

Name: Mr Kenneth Macdonald
Age: 56 years
Occupation: Baker

Prior to this current problem of difficulty in breathing this man has enjoyed good health for many years. Past medical problems have included an appendectomy and a diagnosis of high blood pressure six months previously, for which his GP initially started treatment with bendrofluazide 2.5 mg once daily. But when the blood pressure was checked three months later it was still elevated and the GP decided to add atenolol 100 mg once daily. The blood pressure is now well controlled but for the last three months there has been progressively worsening shortness of breath which is particularly debilitating in the morning. There is an associated cough but no sputum. There has been no weight loss or night sweats.

The gentleman has never smoked and drinks 2–3 pints of beer per week. He runs a small family owned bakery and has indeed worked in the same bakery for nearly 40 years. He lives with his wife and four daughters. Two of the daughters work in the bakery also and have not noticed any respiratory problems. Family history includes the death of his father of a stroke aged 72 years but mother is still alive. There is no other family history of note. There are no known allergies.

He is worried about the possibility of having developed asthma, which may get worse and as a consequence the family business may suffer.

Data gathering in the interview

- Greet the patient and introduce yourself.
- Explain to the patient that his GP referred him with shortness of breath. Invite him to tell you in his own words what the problem is. Ask about any relieving or exacerbating factors for his symptoms and enquire about any diurnal variation in the symptoms. Is there an associated cough and if so is it productive? Are there any constitutional symptoms? Also enquire about any orthopnea and episodes of paroxysmal nocturnal dyspnoea. Does he suffer with a wheeze and has there been any haemoptysis?
- Past medical history. Ask specifically about any previous history of breathing problems. Has he ever been admitted to hospital or been ventilated? Are there any other features of atopy (e.g. eczema, rhinitis)?
- Drug history and allergies.
- Take the social history. Is he a smoker? What is the occupation and is there a chance that it may be responsible for the symptoms (e.g. do the symptoms deteriorate at work)? What impact are the symptoms having on his work? Does he have any pets/birds?
- Ask about any history of illness in the family.
- Make the systems enquiry.
- Now confirm that the information is correct and create a problem list and a possible management plan.

Discussion related to the case

It is crucial that the candidate elicits the history of shortness of breath associated with the commencement of atenolol. This and the fact that the breathing is particularly bothersome in the morning are strongly suggestive of asthma, which is likely to have been exacerbated by the commencement of the B-blocker. Occupational asthma secondary to working as a baker is unlikely, as he has been doing the same job for 40 years; however, it is important that this possibility is raised during the discussion. As a non-smoker, chronic obstructive pulmonary disease is an unlikely proposal. There are no obvious features or risk factors of heart failure, but it must be considered in the differential diagnosis when the shortness of breath occurs in association with the commencement of a beta-blocker.

The candidate should be able to elicit the fact that the patient is concerned about his business and have an idea of what sort of impact the condition is having on the man being able to undertake his work.

Investigations

Investigations should include the following.

- A thorough clinical evaluation of the patient including examination of any sputum and measuring peak expiratory flow rates (PEFR). Say that you would give the patient a diary to take away to monitor PEFR and symptoms. This needs to be done a few times a day to pick up any diurnal variations.
- A chest X-ray review is mandatory and if the recent X-ray requested by the GP is not accessible, another should be requested.
- Spirometry. FEV1/FVC is reduced and residual volume is increased suggesting air trapping. Measurements need to be taken both before and after the administration of a bronchodilator, to assess any reversibility.

Management

You should be familiar with the treatment of asthma and for the latest recommendations refer to the British Thoracic Society web page.

CASE 7: SWOLLEN LEG

Candidate information

You are reviewing patients in the medical admissions unit. Your next patient has been referred by her general practitioner with the following letter. Please read the letter and then review the patient.

Dear Doctor,

Re: Ms Josephine Wilcox

Age: 46 years

This pleasant secretary presented to clinic today with pain and swelling in her left calf. I'm concerned that this may be a DVT. I would be grateful if you would review her and advise on the need for anticoagulation. Your help is greatly appreciated.

Yours sincerely

Subject/Patient's information

Name: Ms Josephine Wilcox
Age: 46 years
Occupation: Secretary

This lady presented to her GP complaining of left leg swelling.

One month ago she returned from an uneventful package holiday in Barcelona. Two weeks later she noticed that her left leg was swollen. The swelling was most prominent below the knee, but there was discernible swelling above the knee also and was associated with a dull ache. Also noticeable was a small amount of bruising on the skin. At this stage she decided to seek medical advice, which has led to the referral today.

Prior to this episode she had been fit and well and does not take any medication, does not smoke or drink alcohol and works as a secretary. She normally lives with her two children and is divorced, hence is the sole breadwinner for the family.

Mrs Wilcox has always been of slim build and although there has been no change in weight, she has noticed that her trousers and skirts have become a bit tight over the abdomen. She has also noticed an irregularity in her periods and 'spotting' between periods. This is unusual for her and she is considering the possibility of this marking the onset of her menopause. Additionally, over the last few months she has noticed a distinct lack of energy and again considers this a possible menopausal symptom.

Data gathering in the interview

- Greet the patient and introduce yourself.
- Explain to the patient that his GP referred has referred her with swelling of the leg and invite her to give you more details on when she noticed the swelling and whether there are any concomitant symptoms. Specifically ask about any shortness of breath and chest pain to consider the possibility of a pulmonary embolus. Ask about any trauma to the leg or associated pain in the knee or hip. Pick up any cues, and if the patient mentions abdominal swelling or the change in periods, then you must follow this up and get further details.
- Past medical history. Is there any past history of thrombosis?
- Drug history and allergies. Specifically ask about the oral contraceptive pill.
- Take the social history. In the context of the presenting complaint it is not enough to simply say that the patient works as a secretary; ask about how many hours she spends at the desk each day, does she get some exercise intermittently etc.
- Ask about any history of illness in the family and make a special enquiry about any family members who have suffered with illnesses associated with a thrombotic tendency (DVT, PE, strokes etc).
- Make the systems enquiry.
- Now confirm that the information is correct and create a problem list and a possible management plan.

Discussion related to the case

The differential diagnoses for a swollen leg are shown Table 1. The examiners will expect to work systematically through this list and come up with the most likely diagnosis. A venous thrombus is more likely than an infectious aetiology such as cellulitis as with the latter we would expect some degree of systemic symptoms suggestive of sepsis (fever, lethargy), which are not present in this case. The ruptured Baker's cyst tends to cause swelling behind the knee is often asymptomatic but may give rise to pain. Mechanical trauma is unlikely as there has been no injury and lymphatic obstruction would cause gradual swelling of the whole leg. So the most likely diagnosis is a deep vein thrombosis.

TABLE 1 Causes of a swollen leg

- Deep vein thrombosis (DVT).
- Thrombophlebitis.
- Cellulitis.
- Ruptured Baker's cyst (history of arthritis may be present).
- Mechanical: trauma, sprain, etc.
- Lymphatic obstruction (pelvic tumour, lymph node enlargement).

Deep vein thrombosis (DVT)

The risk factors for venous thromboembolic disease were first recognised by Virchow and described as the *Virchow's Triad*: venous stasis, hyper-coagulability, and vessel wall injury. Specific risk factors that are worth considering when taking the medical history should include the following:

- **Immobility**, which leads to venous stasis. Causes of immobility may include recent surgery or injury and obviously older age. Immobility during long haul flights is often quoted as a risk factor for the development of a DVT. Obesity is considered a potential risk factors but it may be because morbidly obese people are less mobile than thinner people.
- **Malignancy.** This is a significant risk factor and occult malignancy should be suspected in any patient presenting with a DVT. Hence in this patient it is imperative to follow the lead on the abdominal swelling and irregular menses to consider the possibility of a gynaecological malignancy.
- **Surgery and anaesthesia** are recognised as independent risk factors.
- **Pills and pregnancy.** Oral contraceptive pills increase the risk of venous thromboembolism and pulmonary emboli are the biggest cause of non-traumatic death during pregnancy.
- **Miscellaneous conditions.** SLE, IBD, polycythaemia, thrombocytosis and hyperlipidaemia are just some of the conditions associated with an increased risk of developing a DVT.

- **Coagulopathies.** It is worth considering the possibility of coagulopathies resulting in a hypercoagulable state, particularly when confronted with a younger patient with a recurrent DVT. Important ones include Protein C, Protein S, or antithrombin III deficiencies, antiphospholipid syndrome and activated Protein C (APC) resistance. The commonest, however, (approximately 5% of the UK population) is the carriage of the factor V Leiden gene. This is a single point mutation resulting in a five-fold increase in the risk of developing a DVT.

Investigations

Tell the examiners that first and foremost you would clinically assess the patient, particularly looking for (and measuring) obvious asymmetry between the two legs and looking for signs of infection. In this particular patient it is important also to examine the abdomen to look for evidence of pathology (presence of a mass, ascites or lymph nodes). Blood tests to be considered include a full blood count (to look for evidence of polycythaemia and thrombocytosis) and a D-dimer, which is usually elevated with a blood clot. Duplex ultrasonography with colour Doppler studies is the initial diagnostic modality in most hospitals but may falsely fail to diagnose a DVT in approximately one-third of the patients. Venography is more sensitive but is much more time consuming and requires a skilful operator and also can result in a false negative. Magnetic resonance venography may be the choice of the future, as this can be as sensitive as contrast venography but less invasive and will often give an alternative diagnosis when the cause of the leg swelling is not a DVT. In the context of the clinical history, this lady should also have imaging of the abdomen either with an ultrasound scan or a CT.

Management

The mainstay of management for a DVT is anticoagulation. These days this is usually achieved initially with subcutaneous fractionated low molecular weight heparins and long term with warfarin. It is important to note that warfarin reduces the levels of anticoagulants before reducing procoagulant proteins and hence induces a hypercoagulable state in the first few days, which may worsen the thrombosis. Hence warfarin should only be commenced after heparin.

CASE 8: PALPITATIONS

Candidate information

You are reviewing patients in the medical outpatient clinic. Your next patient has been referred by her general practitioner with the following letter. Please read the letter and then review the patient.

Dear Doctor,

Re: Ms Katrina Fry

Age: 24 years

Thank you for your opinion on this young lady who has presented to the clinic on two occasions complaining of palpitations, associated with chest pain and breathing difficulties. On both of these occasions the duration of her symptoms were short lived and she was well when she arrived in the consulting rooms. She tends to drink a lot of coffee and I suspect this is the cause but still your opinion on excluding more serious pathology would be appreciated.

Yours sincerely

P.S. Unfortunately our ECG machine is broken so I was unable to forward tracing today.

Subject/Patient's information

Name: Ms Katrina Fry
Age: 24 years
Occupation: Advertising executive

This lady has experienced a severe pounding in her chest on a few occasions over the past 12 months, which have become very severe on the last two occasions, prompting her to seek medical advice. Also worrying has been associated shortness of breath and chest discomfort. These episodes have been precipitated by exercise but have been self-limiting, usually lasting for a few minutes. The episodes have never resulted in the loss of consciousness. There has been no associated weight loss or a change in the bowel habit and she has not noticed any heat intolerance or excessive sweating. There are no headaches or visual disturbances.

She has previously been fit and has never been admitted to hospital although as a young woman she was diagnosed as bulimic and required treatment by a psychiatrist. She was also diagnosed with asthma 10 years previously and uses a salbutamol inhaler occasionally (approximately once per week), and is not taking any other regular medications.

She drinks about three bottles of red wine each week and smokes 15 cigarettes a day and has about seven cups of coffee each day. Lives with her younger sister. Her father died in his forties of an acute myocardial infarction but mother is alive and well and lives with her second husband.

Data gathering in the interview
- Greet the patient and introduce yourself.
- Invite her to tell you about the symptoms that have prompted her present referral. Does it sound like a genuine episode of palpitations or is an anxiety attack more likely? Is there any obvious precipitant? How long does each episode last and what tends to terminate it? Is she able to tap out a rate and is it regular or irregular?
- Past medical history. Are there any features of or a previous diagnosis of thyrotoxicosis?
- Drug history and allergies. Is she taking any drugs that may be pro-arrhythmic?
- Take the social history. It is very important to take a detailed history on consumption of caffeine (coffee, tea, soft drinks). Also enquire about smoking and alcohol.
- Family history. Is there a history of sudden collapse or even death in the family?
- Make the systems enquiry.
- Now confirm that the information is correct and create a problem list and a possible management plan.

Discussion related to the case
There is a wide differential diagnosis in this young lady who presents with new onset palpitations (*see* Table 2). The aetiology may be benign (e.g. ectopic activity) or simply related to her consumption of alcohol,

cigarettes and caffeine. Although beta-agonists such as salbutamol may causes palpitations, this lady only uses her inhaler once weekly and it would be a very unlikely cause.

TABLE 2 Causes of palpitations

Psychiatric	• Anxiety and panic disorders.
Cardiac causes	*Arrhythmias:* • sinus tachycardia • bradyarrhythmias (e.g. sick sinus syndrome) • ectopic or premature beats • atrial fibrillation or flutter • supraventricular tachycardia • Wolff-Parkinson-White syndrome • ventricular tachycardia. *Non-arrhythmias:* • congenital heart disease • valvular disease including mitral valve prolapse • congestive cardiac failure • cardiomyopathy • pericarditis • atrial or ventricular septal defects • overactive pacemaker.
Non cardiac causes	• fever. • anaemia. • hyperthyroidism. • electrolyte imbalance. • hypoglycaemia. • phaeochromocytoma. • vasovagal syndrome.
Drugs	• caffeine. • alcohol. • tobacco. • cocaine. • prescription medicines, e.g. salbutamol, thyroxine, theophylline, phenothiazine etc.

Baseline investigations should include:

- Blood tests: FBC to look for anaemia, UE, any electrolyte disturbances? Ruling out hyperkalaemia is particularly important, TFT.
- ECG: May confirm an arrhythmia. Other important considerations include heart block, left or right ventricular hypertrophy, atrial enlargement, short PR interval and delta waves (Wolff-Parkinson-White syndrome), or prolonged QT interval.

Further investigations that may be considered include 24 hour ECG monitoring and cardiac echocardiography to look for evidence of valvular heart disease.

The commonest finding on ambulatory monitoring is benign atrial or ventricular ectopic beats associated with normal sinus rhythm and management constitutes simple appropriate patient education. However, specialist care may be necessary with sustained and more sinister arrhythmias, the management being tailored to the underlying diagnosis. Occasionally, clinical evaluation and diagnostic testing fail to reveal any abnormality or aetiology for the palpitations. These individuals should be advised to abstain from or avoid potential triggers, e.g. caffeine, alcohol, stress.

CASE 9: LOSS OF LIBIDO

Candidate information

You are reviewing patients in the medical outpatient clinic. Your next patient has been referred by his general practitioner with the following letter. Please read the letter and then review the patient.

Dear Doctor,

Re: Mr Rupert Latham

Age: 47 years

Many thanks for seeing this chap who has noted loss of his libido. He is a heterosexual man and tells me that previously he has always enjoyed a 'healthy' sex life. His only past medical history is of diet controlled diabetes. Recent routine blood tests were all normal except a very mild transaminitis. He admits to drinking three pints of beer each day. Many thanks for your help.

Yours sincerely

Subject/Patient's information

Name: Mr Rupert Latham
Age: 47 years
Occupation: Documentary filmmaker

Over the past six months, this gentleman has noticed a reduction in his libido and now rarely has any sexual drive. He is able to have an erection, which occurs spontaneously in the morning but is not associated with sexual desire. This has led to relationship problems with his wife, who has accused Mr Latham of loss of interest in her. Previously, they enjoyed sexual intercourse 3–4 times per week over a 20-year marriage.

Furthermore, he has been suffering lethargy pains in his joints, particularly the knees. On some days he doesn't feel up to getting out of bed. The past medical history is unremarkable except for a diagnosis of diet controlled diabetes mellitus in the past year. He is not taking any regular medication and has no known allergies. He smokes the occasional cigar and tends to drink 2–3 pints of beer each evening.

Mr Latham's father died in a vehicle accident at the age of 38 years but his mother is alive and well. He has one sister aged 42 years who is also well.

Data gathering in the interview

- Greet the patient and introduce yourself.
- Invite him to tell you about his medical problems. The gentleman may find it very difficult to talk about his sexual problems and hence you may need to prompt him further. Pick up on non-verbal cues. It is important that information is gleaned which shows that this is not an erectile dysfunction (impotence) and that there is genuine loss of libido or sexual desire.
- Past medical history. Enquire about the duration of the diabetes and whether it was associated with nerve damage/neuropathy. Take a detailed rheumatological history when the patient describes the pain in the knees.
- Drug history and allergies. It may be worth asking specifically about drugs known to affect sexual desire (*see* Table 3).
- Take the social history. Alcohol is well known to cause loss of libido and people will often be quite guarded about consumption so be sure to take a detailed history quantifying the number of units consumed each week.
- Family history.
- Make the systems enquiry.
- Now confirm that the information is correct and create a problem list and a possible management plan.

Discussion related to the case

Loss of libido is much less common in men compared to women and, if it is a persistent problem, requires formal evaluation and if necessary investigation and treatment. Possible causes are shown in Table 3.

When assessing this gentleman, important questions to ask include: Is this man complaining of an erectile dysfunction or loss of sexual interest with normal erectile function? Hence, it is imperative that you establish that the man is able to achieve an erection. Is this an organic problem or a psychiatric one?

This man seems to be suffering with a genuine loss of libido with normal erectile function. This coupled with the other clues of abnormal liver biochemistry, joint pain, lethargy and the recent diagnosis lead us to the possible diagnosis of hereditary haemochromatosis.

Genetic or primary haemochromatosis is an iron-storage disorder where there is an inappropriate increase in the absorption of iron from the gut. This excess iron is deposited in various organs (heart, liver, pancreas and the pituitary gland) and joints, leading to symptoms. The condition is inherited as an autosomal recessive trait affecting 1 in 300 of the Caucasian population. Symptoms include skin pigmentation, arthritis, diabetes, hepatomegaly, cardiac failure and lethargy.

TABLE 3 Possible causes of loss of libido in men

- Normal part of the aging process.
- Psychological causes: depression and relationship problems.
- Alcohol abuse.
- Drugs: antihypertensives
  - hyperprolactinaemic drugs in men (e.g. phenothiazines, haloperidol)
  - anti-androgenic drugs in men (e.g. cimetidine, finasteride).
- Hypothalamic/pituitary disease.
- Renal failure.
- Adrenal failure.
- Primary testicular disease.

Investigations

Investigations should include serum ferritin and transferrin saturation (serum iron/TIBC). If these suggest iron overload, a liver biopsy should be undertaken which demonstrates marked parenchymal iron deposition with iron staining of the tissue. The hepatic iron concentration and the hepatic iron index (hepatic iron concentration/age) are the most helpful in distinguishing genetic haemochromatosis from the increased iron overload that is seen in other chronic liver diseases.

Management

Management involves the removal of excess body iron (by regular vene-section) and supportive treatment of the damaged organs. Patients are at risk of developing liver failure and hepatocellular carcinoma and should be followed by a gastroenterologist, unless the disease is diagnosed at an early stage. First-degree relatives should be screened for the condition.

CASE 10: DYSPHAGIA

Candidate information

You are reviewing patients in the medical outpatient clinic. Your next patient has been referred by his general practitioner with the following letter. Please read the letter and then review the patient.

Dear Doctor,

Re: Mr Phillip Pattison

Age: 73 years

Thank you for seeing this fellow who has been complaining of heartburn for some months. He has had some problems with swallowing. Please advise whether he requires an endoscopy. Thank you.

Yours sincerely

Subject/Patient's information

Name: Mr Phillip Pattison
Age: 73 years
Occupation: Retired university lecturer

This gentleman has been suffering with intermittent heartburn for most of his adult life, and over the years has self medicated with over-the-counter remedies. His symptoms have deteriorated over the last six months, and now he is having trouble swallowing both liquids and solids. This has resulted in weight loss of approximately half a stone.

The past medical history is unremarkable except for long-standing hypertension treated with an ACE inhibitor. He is an ex-smoker, having given up 11 years ago, and tends to drink a bottle of wine at the weekends. He is an only child and doesn't have any significant family history. He lives with his wife and they have two grown up daughters, who are extremely well.

Data gathering in the interview

- Greet the patient and introduce yourself.
- Tell the patient that his GP has referred him with swallowing difficulties and invite him to give you a personal account of his symptoms. It is important to get an idea of whether the dysphagia is related to liquids, solids or both. Ask about weight loss and attempt to quantify this. He will probably mention his history of long-standing 'heartburn' and ask about the frequency of symptoms (daily, weekly or less frequent).
- Past medical history. Has he previously had an upper GI endoscopy or a barium swallow study?
- Drug history and allergies. Is he on any antacids (prescription or over-the-counter)?
- Take the social history. Both alcohol and cigarette smoking are recognised independent risk factors for the development of oesophageal squamous carcinoma and oesophageal adenocarcinoma (by perhaps increasing the risk of gastro-oesophageal reflux disease, GORD).
- Ask about any history of illness in the family.
- Make the systems enquiry.
- Now confirm that the information is correct and create a problem list and a possible management plan.

Discussion related to the case

There are numerous causes of dysphagia, as shown in Table 4. These can be classified on the basis of the diagnosis as shown in the table or perhaps more arbitrarily on the basis of patient's subjective level of dysphagia, either as high or low dysphagia. High dysphagia is caused by neurological conditions (e.g. CVA, bulbar palsy) or ENT conditions (e.g. pharyngeal pouch, malignancy). Low dysphagia tends to be due to oesophageal disease. In clinical practice it is often difficult to differentiate high dysphagia from globus hystericus. Globus often affects young people, where there is a feeling of a 'lump in the throat' without true dysphagia and investigations prove to be unremarkable. Although it is often associated with gastro-oesophageal reflux disease, it is generally considered to be a benign 'functional' disorder.

While taking the history it is crucial to get as much detail as possible about the duration and nature of the dysphagia. For instance, patients with neuromuscular disorder may find it harder to swallow liquids (and experience nasal regurgitation) compared with solid or semi-solid diets.

Patients with achalasia have a long duration of dysphagia to both liquids and solids, without associated weight loss.

Investigations and management

As a general rule, elderly patients with new onset dysphagia and associated weight loss should be considered high risk for upper GI malignancy and investigated promptly with a gastroscopy. This gentleman fits this category and warrants an urgent gastroscopy. Particularly as he has a long standing history of gastro-oesophageal reflux disease, a recognised risk factor for oesophageal adenocarcinoma which is often preceded by the development of Barrett's oesophagus. If cancer is confirmed, staging can be undertaken with CT scanning and, for smaller tumours, endoscopic ultrasound scanning may be appropriate.

TABLE 4 Causes of dysphagia

Obstructive	• oesophagitis
	• oesophageal cancer
	• benign oesophageal stricture/web
	• gastric cancer
	• ENT cancer.
Neurological	• stroke
	• achalasia
	• diffuse oesophageal spasm
	• motor neurone disease
	• Parkinson's and other degenerative disorder
	• myasthenia gravis
	• multiple sclerosis
	• myopathy (e.g. myotonic dystrophy)
	• Chagas disease.
Others	• pharyngeal pouch
	• globus hystericus
	• external compression (e.g. mediastinal tumour, or associated with cervical spondylosis)
	• scleroderma.

Management depends upon confirmation of cancer and the stage. Often the cancer is at an advanced stage at the time of diagnosis and only palliative treatment can be offered. Curative treatment is with surgical resection (usually oesophagectomy), sometimes with adjuvant chemo-therapy and radiotherapy. Palliative treatment may entail re-canalisation of the oesophagus with a metal stent or by tumour ablation with a laser or with an argon plasma coagulator (APC).

CASE 11: UNEXPLAINED WEIGHT LOSS

Candidate information

You are reviewing patients in the medical outpatient clinic. Your next patient has been referred by her general practitioner with the following letter. Please read the letter and then review the patient.

Dear Doctor,

Re: Miss Julie Ross

Age: 26 years

I would greatly value your opinion regarding this young lady who has lost two stone in weight over the past year. She is not on a diet. Routine blood tests were requested but unfortunately have been lost. Please accept my apologies for this.

Yours sincerely

Subject/Patient's information

Name: Miss Julie Ross
Age: 26 years
Occupation: Office worker

This young lady has noticed a weight loss of approximately 2 stone over the course of nine months. Her usual weight is 10 stone, which has now dropped to 8 stone and is concerned particularly as her family and friends often comment on how thin she looks. There has been no discernible change in her appetite, which consists of three regular meals and often desserts and frequent snacks, which include chocolates and crisps. She has not suffered with polydipsia or polyuria but has been suffering with loose stools, which is unusual for her. In the last few months she has become intolerant to heat and has found her office stifling and had complained about the air conditioning not working but no fault had been discovered. The heat had caused her heart to race, causing palpitations. However, she had noticed her heart 'racing' at other times also, particularly at night when trying to sleep. The other noticeable feature has been less frequent and lighter periods.

There is past history of tonsillectomy (aged 12 years) and migraine. She does not take any regular medication, including over the counter medicines and she is not aware of any allergies. She smokes 10 cigarettes a day and dinks 10 'alcopops' over the weekend. Works in an office distributing language courses. She has not been in a relationship for over a year since breaking up with her last boyfriend and has not had any sexual relations over this period. She lives alone in rented accommodation and does not have any pets. There is no family history of serious illness.

Data gathering in the interview
- Greet the patient and introduce yourself.
- Ask the patient to tell you about her medical problems. Keep the questions open to begin with but then go on to get more specific details. Ask her to quantify the amount of weight lost and confirm that she has not been dieting. It is always a good idea to take a detailed history of her daily diet, starting with breakfast, and the examiners will be impressed if you try to work out the approximate calories consumed during the day. Also ask about exercise and whether there has been change in this. Enquire about her bowel habit (diarrhoea? steatorrhoea?). Ask about her opinion of her body in an attempt to gauge any underlying psychiatric co-morbidity.
- Past medical history. Ask about any history of diabetes and thyroid disease. Does she suffer with any other autoimmune conditions?
- Drug history and allergies. Enquire about any new medicines she may have started taking and also ask about any over the counter medicines. Is she taking thyroxine or laxatives?
- Take the social history. What impact are her symptoms having on her work?
- Ask about any history of illness in the family.
- Make the systems enquiry.
- Now confirm that the information is correct and create a problem list and a possible management plan.

Discussion related to the case
A good candidate should be able to take a detailed history of the weight

loss and consider all the potential diagnoses (*see* Table 5). They should also be able to record a comprehensive dietary history and explore any associated symptoms. It is worth knowing that certain conditions cause a profound weight loss with a normal appetite. These include diabetes mellitus, thyrotoxicosis, malabsorption and a phaeochromocytoma.

The constellation of symptoms in this young lady is suggestive of a thyrotoxicosis, which is probably autoimmune in origin (Graves' disease). However, other possible diagnosis cannot be excluded without further investigations.

Investigations
Investigations should include the following.
- Blood tests:
  - FBC
  - UE
  - LFT
  - inflammatory markers (ESR, CRP)
  - anti-endomysial antibody and TTG antibody
  - fasting glucose and OGTT
  - thyroid function tests.
- Endoscopy with duodenal biopsies.

If these tests fail to give the diagnosis, further investigations to identify other potential causes of weight loss may be warranted.

Management
Management depends upon the diagnosis.

TABLE 5 Causes of unexplained weight loss

- Psychiatric illness: anxiety, depression and eating disorders.
- Malignancy, particularly upper GI.
- Gastrointestinal causes: malabsorption, IBD, diarrhoea and vomiting.
- Endocrine causes: DM, thyrotoxicosis, adrenal insufficiency.
- Drugs: amphetamines, laxatives, thyroxine, smoking, cannabis.
- Miscellaneous: phaeochromocytoma, infective (e.g. HIV, TB, parasites).

CASE 12: RENAL IMPAIRMENT

Candidate information

You are reviewing patients in the medical outpatient clinic. Your next patient has been referred by his general practitioner with the following letter. Please read the letter and then review the patient.

Dear Doctor,

Re: Mr Manoj Patel

Age: 48 years

Many thanks for seeing this gentleman who recently had some blood tests which have been found to be abnormal with renal impairment (urea 22, creatinine 218 and haemoglobin 9.6, random serum glucose 12.6). I would be grateful if you would advise on further management.

Yours sincerely,

Subject/Patient's information

Name: Mr Manoj Patel
Age: 48 years
Occupation: Bus driver

This gentleman presented to his GP four weeks previously complaining of lethargy, headaches and anorexia. Subsequent blood tests showed significant renal impairment and anaemia. He has not noticed a decrease in urine output. He is known to suffer with hypertension for many years and has previously been started on a diuretic and an ACE inhibitor to control his blood pressure, but has failed to do so adequately. In all honesty, Mr Patel often neglects to take his tablets.

Six weeks previously he suffered with back pains (which he attributed to his profession) and took his wife's ibuprofen tablets for a week and the symptoms settled. He has no known allergies, is not a smoker or a drinker and works as a bus driver, which he finds tedious.

There is no family history to note, both parents and three siblings are alive and well. He lives with his wife and three children, who are also well.

Data gathering in the interview

- Greet the patient and introduce yourself.
- Tell him that his GP has referred him with concerns regarding his kidneys and ask him to tell you about his medical problems. Begin with open questions followed up with closed, more detailed questioning. Are there any symptoms to suggest he is uraemic: lethargy, pruritis, and nausea? Is he likely to be fluid overloaded (breathlessness, decreased urine output, oedema)?
- Past medical history. Has he previously been diagnosed with renal impairment? Get details of the past medical history of hypertension: when it was diagnosed, what the reading is normally, whether it is controlled by the medication and indeed whether he takes the antihypertensive medication. It is worth asking about any previously diagnosed end organ damage (retinopathy, proteinuria etc). Also enquire if the gentleman has previously been diagnosed with diabetes mellitus. The blood test results on the GP letter certainly indicate that he is a diabetic now.
- Drug history and allergies. Take a detailed drug history, particularly looking for potentially nephrotoxic drugs: NSAIDs, ACEi, diuretics, and certain antibiotics.
- Take the social history.
- Family history. Ask about any history of renal disease (e.g. PCKD) in the family.
- Make the systems enquiry.
- Now confirm that the information is correct and create a problem list and a possible management plan.

Discussion related to the case

A good candidate should be able to take a detailed history from the patient and based on the medical history come up with an idea of the possible causes of the renal failure (*see* Table 6). The candidate should confirm the information with the patient, be able to discuss the implications of the illness on the patient's life (Is he able to continue working as a bus driver?), create a problem list and establish a management plan.

Possible causes of renal failure in this gentleman include hypertensive nephrosclerosis, glomerular disease secondary to diabetes mellitus and drug induced nephropathy. Angiotensin-converting enzyme (ACE) inhibitors and non-steroidal anti-inflammatory drugs (NSAIDs) and diuretics can all cause renal failure, by mechanisms beyond the scope of this present discussion.

Investigations

Investigations for this gentleman may include the following.

- Blood tests.
  - Urea and electrolytes (particularly important to look for hyperkalaemia).
  - Albumin may be low in nephritic syndrome.
  - Serum bicarbonate and calcium may be low while phosphate may be high.
  - FBC to look for evidence of anaemia.
  - C-ANCA (positive in Wegner's granulomatosis) and P-ANCA levels to look for evidence of polyarteritis nodosa or microscopic polyangiitis.
  - Positive anti-glomerular basement membrane (anti-GBM) antibodies are very suggestive of underlying Goodpasture's syndrome.
  - Although unlikely, systemic lupus erythematosus (SLE) can be screened for using antinuclear antibodies (ANA) and double-stranded DNA antibody levels.
  - Serum complement (C3, C4) levels may drop with glomerular disease.
  - HIV, hepatitis B and C and syphilis serology. These tests should not be carried out routinely but may be considered if no other cause for the symptoms can be found.
- Urinalysis and microscopy. Proteinuria points towards tubulointerstitial or glomerular disease. RBC casts are suggestive of a proliferative glomerulonephritis while WBC casts point towards an infective aetiology.
- 24-hour protein excretion and creatinine clearance.
- Radiological tests.
  - Plain abdominal film to look for nephrocalcinosis or radio-opaque stones.
  - Renal ultrasound to look for obvious structural (shrunken kidneys, APCKD, tumour or mass) or obstruction.

- Intravenous urogram (IVU) is not typically performed, as there is potential for contrast-induced nephrotoxicity.
- Radionuclide scans may show evidence of renal artery stenosis.
- CT/MRI where more detailed renal imaging is desirable.

● **Renal biopsy** should be considered if the diagnosis remains elusive.

TABLE 6 Causes of chronic renal failure

Primary glomerular disease	● Minimal change, membranous, Berger's (or IgA) disease, focal segmental glomerulosclerosis (FSGS), membranoproliferative glomerulonephritis, rapidly progressive (crescentic) glomerulonephritis.
Secondary glomerular disease	● Common conditions causing glomerular disease include diabetes mellitus, rheumatological conditions (rheumatoid arthritis, SLE, mixed connective tissue disease, scleroderma), Goodpasture's syndrome, Wegener's granulomatosis, mixed cryoglobulinemia, infections (hepatitis B and C, HIV, syphilis, parasites), drugs (gold, penicillamine, heroin), amyloidosis, light chain deposition disease, neoplasia, haemolytic-uraemic syndrome (HUS), Henoch-Schönlein purpura, Alport syndrome, reflux nephropathy, TTP.
Vascular disease	● Renal artery stenosis, vasculitis (C-ANCA and P-ANCA positive), hypertensive nephrosclerosis, renal vein thrombosis.
Tubulointerstitial disease	● Secondary to drugs (e.g., allopurinol), infections, Sjögren's syndrome, multiple myeloma metabolic disorders (chronic hypokalaemia or hypercalcaemia) sarcoidosis, cystinosis, heavy metals, radiation, polycystic kidneys.
Obstructive uropathy	● Prostatism, renal calculi, malignancy, retroperitoneal fibrosis, urethral stricture.

Management

Management very much depends upon the underlying cause and should be supervised by a specialist. As a general rule, hypertension should be controlled aggressively as should glycaemic control. Any nephrotoxic drugs should be avoided. The patient should be seen by an experienced dietician to control phosphate and potassium intake and should avoid becoming fluid overloaded. Oral phosphate binders, calcium (and possibly calcitriol and vitamin D) may be prescribed. Anaemia may be treated with erythropoietin. Loop diuretics may help with volume overload. The renal function should be monitored closely and replacement therapy (i.e. dialysis) needs to be initiated in a timely fashion. Where appropriate the patient can be considered for a renal transplant.

CASE 13: RECURRENT CHEST INFECTIONS

Candidate information

You are reviewing patients in the medical outpatient clinic. Your next patient has been referred by his general practitioner with the following letter. Please read the letter and then review the patient.

Dear Doctor,

Re: Mr Rupert Wise

Age: 18 years

I would very grateful for your advice on this young lad who has been troubled with repeated chest infections over some time, which seem to be progressively worsening. He is producing copious amounts of purulent sputum and a recent culture has grown a strain of pseudomonas. Clinical examination shows a thin man with obvious finger clubbing. I have tried a number of antibiotics with no success and frankly am now at my wits' end. Once again thank you for your help.

Yours sincerely

Subject/Patient's information

Name: Mr Rupert Wise
Age: 18 years
Occupation: Student

This young man has been suffering with chest infections ever since he can remember, but the situation is progressively worsening and now has reached the stage where he is finding it difficult to cope with his daily symptoms. There seems to be constant production of sputum, which has been tinged with blood on occasions. This is worst first thing in the morning and is associated with a 'hacking' cough and on occasions a wheeze.

Over the years he has been prescribed many courses of antibiotics and multiple inhalers, which have been useful but less so now. As a child he had been referred to a paediatrician who thought it likely that he was suffering with bronchiectasis but the family moved town and did not receive an appointment with another doctor. The past medical history is otherwise unremarkable except for an operation for nasal polyps three years previously.

He lives with his mother and one sister aged 16 years who are both well apart from bouts of depressions that his mother suffers with. The father had been an alcoholic and had abandoned the family when Rupert was four years old. He has not seen his father since. There are no known allergies. He is a non-smoker and rarely drinks alcohol. Currently he is at college working towards a diploma in catering.

Data gathering in the interview
- Greet the patient and introduce yourself.
- Ask the patient to tell you about his medical problems. Find out if there are times of the day when the respiratory problems are worse than others. What is the colour of the sputum and has he ever noticed any blood? Are there any exacerbating or relieving factors? Has he had any courses of antibiotics and have they been helpful?
- Past medical history. Enquire into the past history of respiratory infections. It would be pertinent to ask about any history of whooping cough.
- Drug history and allergies. Is he on any medication and are they helping with his symptoms?
- Take the social history. Be sure to ask about smoking even though he is very young.
- Ask about any history of illness in the family.
- Make the systems enquiry. As there is a suspicion that this could be cystic fibrosis, it would be appropriate to ask about other systems that may be involved. You could specifically ask about any steatorrhoea, abdominal pain and weight loss (as the pancreas and the biliary system can be involved in this condition).
- Now confirm that the information is correct and create a problem list and a possible management plan.

Discussion related to the case
The candidate should be able to take a detailed history from the young man to get insight into his respiratory problems. He/she should be

able to gauge the impact the symptoms have on the man's life, create a problem list and have an investigation and management plan ready.

Recurrent chest infections, copious sputum and finger clubbing are strongly suggestive of a suppurative lung disease such as bronchiectasis. Possible causes include post infection (e.g. measles, pertussis, pneumonia), hypogammaglobulinaemia and cystic fibrosis. Cystic fibrosis usually presents in neonates and infants but can present in adolescents and even young adults.

Investigations

Investigations should include the following.

- Blood tests:
  - FBC, to see if the white cell count is elevated
  - immunoglobulins
  - LFTs and albumin.
- Chest X-ray.
- Sputum microbiology.
- Sweat sodium or chloride concentration measurements on at least two occasions.

Management

In the first instance management should include antibiotics and physio-therapy. Bronchodilators may be helpful if there is a degree of reversibility. Other treatment may be necessary if the diagnosis confirms cystic fibrosis (see below).

Cystic fibrosis (CF)

This is possibly the most common (1:2500) lethal, autosomal recessive inherited condition in Caucasians. End stage lung disease is the principle cause of death. One in 25 people are asymptomatic carriers of the gene. Mutations in the gene for cystic fibrosis transmembrane conductance regulator (CFTR) result in abnormalities of chloride transport across mucosal surfaces, leading to increased mucus viscosity. This in turn leads to stagnation, infection and inflammation and chronic damage. Lungs, intestines, pancreas, biliary tree and the vas deferens in males can all be affected. Patients typically present as neonates with meconium ileus or as young children with recurrent respiratory tract infections or symptoms of malabsorption. Investigation is as above and management is symptomatic. This should include lung physiotherapy and antibiotics as required.

CASE 14: ACHES AND PAINS

Candidate information

You are reviewing patients in the medical outpatient clinic. Your next patient has been referred by his general practitioner with the following letter. Please read the letter and then review the patient.

Dear Doctor,

Re: Mr Sylvester Duncan-Thomas

Age: 38 years

Thank you for seeing this interesting chap who presented himself to my surgery last week with 'aches' in his hands and feet. I did notice a faint smell of alcohol on his breath and I did wonder whether he might have gout. I have prescribed him some analgesia but wondered whether he warrants further investigation. Once again thank you for your help.

Yours sincerely

Subject/Patient's information

Name: Mr Sylvester Duncan-Thomas
Age: 38 years
Occupation: Farmer

This gentleman has been suffering with pains in his hand and feet for a few weeks, which has made it difficult to perform manual tasks. Over the counter analgesics have only resulted in a limited improvement of his symptoms, which are becoming progressively worse. The pain is worse first thing in the morning and is associated with stiffness.

His past medical history is unremarkable except for psoriasis, diagnosed five years previously. This tends to affect his elbows and scalp and responds well to topical treatment. Normally, he is not on any other medication and has no known allergies. However, his GP has prescribed ibuprofen 400 mg tid, which seems to be helping with the symptoms.

He doesn't smoke other than a cigar at New Year's Eve. Moreover, he only drinks alcohol very occasionally (probably two pints of beer each month). On the afternoon of the visit to the GP's surgery he had a pint of beer at the annual village fair. He lives with his mother, but has had a steady girlfriend for seven years. His father died at the age of 76 years following a stroke. There is an older sister now living in Portugal who has a history of 'rheumatism'.

Data gathering in the interview
- Greet the patient and introduce yourself.
- Tell the patient that he has been referred by his GP because of pain in his hands and feet and invite him to give you a detailed history. As described previously in Case 2, pay particular attention to symptoms of pain, swelling, stiffness and the degree of disability incurred.
- Past medical history. Has he previously been diagnosed with a rheumatological problem?
- Drug history and allergies. Is he on analgesics (e.g. NSAIDs) and are they helping with the symptoms?
- Take the social history, including a detailed history of alcohol ingestion. What is his vocation and what is the functional consequence of his symptoms?
- Ask about any history of illness in the family.
- Make the systems enquiry.
- Now confirm that the information is correct and create a problem list and a possible management plan.

Discussion related to the case
This case illustrates the importance of keeping an open mind, while reading the referral letter for the patient. In this instance, the judgemental candidate would assume that the patient's problems were related to excess alcohol consumption, which is clearly not the case. The past medical history is very important as it raises the possibility of psoriatic arthritis, although there are other possibilities. Moreover the family history also points to the likely diagnosis of a rheumatological condition.

Psoriatic arthritis is a chronic inflammatory arthritis that develops in 5–40% of patients with psoriasis. It is important to appreciate that the arthritis may precede the skin complaint. The arthritis can present in at least five different forms (*see* Table 7).

Investigations

Diagnosis is generally clinical although blood tests (e.g. inflammatory markers) and joint X-rays may help.

Management

Management generally involves the treatment of underlying symptoms, e.g. with NSAIDs and the treatment of the psoriasis, e.g. with photo-therapy. Occasionally, second line agents such as steroids, cyclosporine, sulfasalazine, methotrexate and infliximab may be necessary.

TABLE 7 Five patterns of psoriatic arthritis

Distal interphalangeal (DIP) arthropathy	• Although considered typical of psoriatic arthritis, in fact it occurs only in 5–10% of patients. There may be marked inflammation of the nail.
Arthritis mutilans	• There is 'telescoping' of the fingers with severe deformity.
Asymmetrical oligoarticular arthritis	• Generally five or fewer joints are affected, often in the hands. Patients typically develop dactylitis with the so-called 'sausage' appearance.
Symmetrical polyarthritis	• The appearances are similar to and indeed may be mistaken for rheumatoid arthritis.
Spondylitis	• This may be associated with sacroiliitis.
Juvenile psoriatic arthritis	• This accounts for up to 20% of childhood arthritis. Onset is around the age of 10 years and in some patients it progresses to a severe debilitating arthritis in adulthood.

CASE 15: DIFFICULT TO TREAT CHEST INFECTION

Candidate information

You are reviewing patients in the medical outpatient clinic. Your next patient has been referred by her general practitioner with the following letter. Please read the letter and then review the patient.

Dear Doctor,

Re: Mrs Eunice Lambert

Age: 61 years

I would very much value your opinion on this delightful lady who has been complaining of shortness of breath, cough and sputum production over the last few months. She has had multiple courses of antibiotics with no real improvement in her symptoms. A chest X-ray was reported as: *hyperinflated lungs, no focal lesion seen*. Despite this I remain concerned and look forward to you advice.

Yours sincerely

Subject/Patient's information

Name: Mrs Eunice Lambert
Age: 61 years
Occupation: Retired school teacher

This lady has been suffering with her shortness of breath and a productive cough for many months. The sputum tends to be yellow and occasionally green but never bloodstained. The cough is worse first thing in the morning. There is no noticeable ankle swelling or worsening of symptoms on lying down flat. The GP has tried a number of different antibiotics, which have failed to improve symptoms to any significant extent. Moreover, he has given her a blue and a brown inhaler that do make a difference. Eunice isn't sure how to use the inhalers properly and simply tends to spray them into her mouth from about 3 inches.

She has been a smoker of 20 cigarettes a day for 42 years and used to drink a glass of sherry most nights until recently. She used to work as a geography teacher in a secondary school, but has been retired for three years. She is unaware of exposure to asbestos or any other hazardous materials or chemicals. She lives with her husband Warren and a pet cat and two canaries.

Data gathering in the interview

- Greet the patient and introduce yourself.
- Explain to the patient that her GP referred her because of the breathing difficulties and invite her to describe her problems. Particularly ask about cough, wheeze and sputum production (Is it copious? Is it bloodstained?). It is also worth enquiring into the possibility of cardiological disease and ask about symptoms of orthopnea and paroxysmal nocturnal dyspnoea.
- Past medical history. Has she ever been hospitalised with chest infections?
- Drug history and allergies. Take a detailed account of all the drugs she is using, including inhalers or nebulisers. At this juncture you should ask about her inhaler technique (remember, the examiners are checking your skill eliciting an accurate medical history and you should not ask the patient to give you a demonstration).
- Take the social history. For obvious reasons, the smoking history is especially important and you should approximate the pack years. Occupational history and documenting potential allergens (such as pets) is essential.
- Ask about any history of illness in the family.
- Make the systems enquiry.
- Now confirm that the information is correct and create a problem list and a possible management plan.

Discussion related to the case

The clinical history is strongly suggestive of a diagnosis of chronic obstructive pulmonary disease (COPD). Late onset asthma is an alternative (but less likely) possibility. NICE guidelines (Feb. 2004) make it clear that there is no single diagnostic test for COPD and that diagnosis is based on a combination of clinical judgement and spirometry to confirm airways obstruction. Airflow obstruction is defined as a FEV1 (forced expiratory volume in 1 second) of less than 80% expected and a

FEV1/FVC ratio less than 0.7. Relevant investigations and management of the condition as suggested by these guidelines is discussed here.

Investigations
All patients should have the following investigations at the time of diagnosis.
- Full blood count to look for evidence of anaemia and poly-cythaemia.
- Chest X-ray.
- Spirometry.

Additional investigations may be performed in certain situations.
- Peak flow rate measurements – to exclude the possibility of asthma if doubt remains.
- Alpha-1-antitrypsin – if the disease seems to be more severe than expected from the smoking history or if there is a family history of illness.
- CT scan – to investigate abnormalities on a chest X-ray.
- ECG and echocardiogram – if there is a suspicion of cor pulmonale.
- Pulse oximetry – to asses the need for oxygen therapy.
- Sputum culture – if the patient is producing purulent sputum and antibiotic therapy needs to be directed to the specific organism.

Management
The key priorities in the management of these patients are as follows.
- **Smoking cessation (and pulmonary rehabilitation).** This is crucial to the subsequent management and prognosis of the condition and every opportunity should be used to help patients quit cigarettes for good. Advice to encourage a healthier lifestyle, e.g. nutrition, exercise, alcohol, should also be given.
- **Effective inhaled therapy.** Technique should be checked before prescribing inhalers.
  - Short-acting and if necessary long-acting inhaled bronchodilators (beta-agonists, e.g. salbutamol and/or anticholinergics, e.g. ipratropium bromide)
  - Inhaled corticosteroids should be added to the long-acting bronchodilators in patients with a FEV1 less than or equal to 50% predicted value, who have had two or more exacerbations in the previous 12 months.

- Nebulisers should be prescribed for patients who remain breathless despite maximal inhaler therapy.
- **Theophyllines** may be used in some patients but caution has to be exercised to avoid toxicity and interactions.
- **Corticosteroids.**
  - Inhaled corticosteroids may be prescribed in patients with a FEV1 less than or equal to 50% predicted, who are having two or more exacerbations requiring treatment with antibiotics or oral corticosteroids in a 12-month period.
  - Oral corticosteroids should be avoided as long-term maintenance therapy and should be restricted to the treatment of acute exacerbations. Where it is necessary to use them long term, prophylaxis should be given to prevent osteoporosis.
- **Management of exacerbations.** Frequency and severity of exacerbations should be reduced with 'self-help' advice, particularly to respond quickly to exacerbations and with the appropriate use of bronchodilators, corticosteroids, antibiotics, vaccinations (e.g. against influenza) and where appropriate non-invasive ventilation.
- **Use non-invasive ventilation (NIV).** Patients with persistent hypercapnic ventilatory failure during exacerbations not responding to medical therapy may require NIV, which should be delivered by trained staff in a specialist unit. Patients who are commenced on NIV should have a clear plan regarding further management, i.e. determine whether they would be appropriate for full ventilatory support.

CASE 16: HEADACHE

Candidate information

You are reviewing patients in the medical outpatient clinic. Your next patient has been referred by her general practitioner with the following letter. Please read the letter and then review the patient.

Dear Doctor,

Re: Mrs Mary McBride

Age: 56 years

Many thanks for seeing this nice lady who has been complaining of a headache for some months and analgesics have only been of limited help. I wonder whether she needs further investigations. Please help.

Yours sincerely

Subject/Patient's information

Name: Mrs Mary McBride
Age: 56 years
Occupation: Secretary

This lady has been suffering with headaches for some months and the GP has now referred her to this clinic for further assessment. The headaches tend to be present first thing in the morning and on occasions have woken her up from sleep. Also more recently she has noticed that coughing, sneezing and bending over all exacerbate the headache. However, the pain is never severe and usually settles of its own accord or with analgesia, which includes codeine phosphate and paracetamol. The codeine tends to constipate her so she takes this only when the pain fails to respond to the paracetamol alone. This was infrequent but now tends to be every other day. There is no nausea or vomiting. She does not take any other medicines and has no known allergies. She smoked briefly as a young woman over 30 years ago and never drinks alcohol, as she dislikes the taste.

After leaving school, Mrs McBride worked in a supermarket but subsequently trained as a secretary and has been working in the offices of a factory manufacturing plastic furniture. She is married with three children. One of her children has learning difficulties and can be very difficult to manage at times and has been a source of some stress over the years. In addition she has had some marital difficulties and is finding it hard to maintain her relationship with her husband. There is no family history of any serious illness and in fact both parents and all four siblings are alive and well.

Data gathering in the interview

- Greet the patient and introduce yourself.
- Explain to the lady that her GP has referred her because of the headaches and invite her to give you an account of when she first noticed the problem. Be sure that she gives details of the duration of the problem, any obvious exacerbating and relieving factors, including the time of the day when the pain is at its worst. Enquire into the extent to which the analgesics are helping and whether there is any nausea or vomiting associated. It is also very important to ask about any visual disturbances and indeed any other prodromal symptoms associated with the pain.
- Past medical history. Specifically ask about any history of hypertension and any trauma that the patient may have suffered. It is also worth asking about her mental well-being, particularly to look for evidence of depression and anxiety.
- Drug history and allergies. Patients that overuse analgesics can get rebound headaches and hence it is important to document doses.
- Take the social history. Withdrawal from drugs such as caffeine, nicotine and alcohol can cause headaches.
- Family history.
- Make the systems enquiry.
- Now confirm that the information is correct and create a problem list and a possible management plan.

Discussion related to the case

Headaches are one of the commonest reasons for patients to seek medical advice. The diagnosis can range from completely benign conditions to those that can be life threatening (*see* Table 8). For this reason, it can be extremely difficult for the doctor to decide on how far the investigations need to be taken. Obviously, it is inappropriate for all patients to undergo radiological imaging (e.g. CT head, MRI) but the consequence of missing severe pathology can be disastrous.

Investigations should be guided by the clinical history and may include blood tests such as an ESR to look for evidence of inflammation, MRI/CT head and lumbar puncture. Management is also guided by the diagnosis.

In this case the history is very suspicious of a raised intracranial pressure. The headache is characteristically present on waking or may even wake the patient from sleep and may be worsened by coughing, sneezing or exertion. Nausea, vomiting, papilloedema, focal neurology may be present, which further suggest intracranial hypertension and imaging should be undertaken as a matter of priority. Lumbar puncture is relatively contraindicated as it may give rise to 'coning'.

TABLE 8 Causes of headaches

Intracranial disease	• e.g. brain tumours, bleeds, infections, benign intracranial hypertension, vascular disorders (e.g. venous sinus thrombosis), obstructive hydrocephalus.
Intracranial disease	• e.g. systemic hypertension, hypoxia (including altitude sickness) and hypercapnia.
Drugs and toxins	• e.g. nitrates, PPIs, rebound from overuse of analgesics, drug withdrawal (e.g. nicotine).
Others	• stress, tension headache, giant cell arteritis, glaucoma, sinusitis, cluster headaches (migrainous neuralgia).

CASE 17: PAINFUL HANDS

Candidate information

You are reviewing patients in the medical outpatient clinic. Your next patient has been referred by her general practitioner with the following letter. Please read the letter and then review the patient.

Dear Doctor,

Re: Mrs Sally O'Sullivan

Age: 32 years

Please advise on the management of this young woman who has developed pain in her hands. There is clear tenderness when examining her hands but there are no convincing features of an arthropathy. The only other abnormalities on clinical inspection are a facial flush and a soft systolic murmur. She has a past history of thrombosis and has previously been on warfarin.

I would therefore greatly value your opinion on how to proceed. Best wishes.

Yours sincerely

Subject/Patient's information

Name: Mrs Sally O'Sullivan
Age: 32 years
Occupation: School catering assistant

This lady presented to her GP complaining of several months' history of pains, predominantly in her fingers, although she has also been suffering with similar aches in her knees and wrists. In addition, she has also noticed intermittent low-grade fevers, anorexia and one stone in weight loss over the past three months. On occasions there has been chest discomfort and a difficulty in breathing. There have also been painful ulcers in the mouth. The only other problem she has noticed is a rash appearing on her cheeks, worsening with sunlight.

Her past medical history includes two miscarriages a few years ago and a deep vein thrombosis in the left calf six months previously for which she received warfarin. Her only medication at present is analgesic drugs including paracetamol and Voltarol (diclofenac) and long-standing cimetidine, for dyspepsia symptoms. She has no known allergies. She has never been on the oral contraceptive pill and is actively trying for a baby with her husband. Her previous miscarriages were not investigated, but she is currently waiting for an appointment to see the obstetrician.

The only family history she can recall is that her mother suffers with an overactive thyroid gland. She does not smoke cigarettes or drink alcohol. Her symptoms are making the job as a catering assistant difficult and she has had to take time off work.

Data gathering in the interview
- Greet the patient and introduce yourself.
- Explain to the lady that her GP has referred her because of the pain in her hands and invite her to give you a detailed account of her symptoms. Refer to Case 2 for details on taking a rheumatological history. Ask about the impact her symptoms have had on her lifestyle. Then enquire about other symptoms the patient may have noticed. Carefully catalogue each and ask brief details in order to formulate a differential diagnosis.
- Past medical history. Has she any past medical history of arthritis? Has she had multiple thromboembolic episodes and has she ever had a miscarriage? Does she suffer with renal impairment?
- Drug history and allergies. In view of the past history of thrombosis, specifically ask about the oral contraceptive pill. Is she on any analgesics and are they helping with her symptoms?
- Take the social history.
- Family history.
- Make the systems enquiry.
- Now confirm that the information is correct and create a problem list and a possible management plan.

Discussion related to the case
There are enough clues in the GP's letter for the candidate to consider the possibility of systemic lupus erythematosus (SLE) and certainly the history is suggestive of this diagnosis. Infective endocarditis is another

possibility in view of the murmur and fever, but the other features are more suggestive of a non-bacterial (Libman-Sacks endocarditis), which is associated with SLE. Moreover, the previous history of thrombophilia point towards a diagnosis of secondary anti-phospholipid syndrome associated with SLE.

Systemic lupus erythematosus (SLE)

SLE is a complex autoimmune disease with multisystem manifestations secondary to the circulating immune complexes and autoantibodies. The American College of Rheumatology has suggested that to make a likely diagnosis of SLE at least four out of the following 11 criteria need to be present:
- malar rash
- discoid rash
- photosensitivity
- oral ulcers
- arthritis
- serositis
- renal disorder
- leucopoenia, haemolytic anaemia, or thrombocytopenia
- neurological disorder
- positive anti-DNA or anti-Sm antibody, or positive test for antiphospholipid antibodies
- antinuclear antibodies positive.

The prevalence of the condition is approximately 0.2%. It is nearly 10 times more common in women and more common (×4) in Blacks/Asians and in pregnancy (and with the oral contraceptive pill). Its peak incidence is in women in their twenties or thirties who are of child-bearing age. Some drugs can produce a lupus-like syndrome. Well-recognised examples with definite association include procainamide, hydralazine, and isoniazid. There are other drugs that may be associated. An example of these includes cimetidine, which our patient in the case above has been taking.

The long-term prognosis of the condition in developed nations is >95% survival at 10 years. Death may be caused by early atherosclerosis (leading to cerebrovascular and cardiovascular disease), renal failure, sepsis and others such as neurological disease.

Symptoms of SLE can be extremely diverse, affecting many different systems. Hence the condition may present under different specialists, perhaps masquerading as another illness. Systems affected include the following.

- **Musculoskeletal:** arthralgia and arthritis, but pain is worse than the physical signs. A deforming arthropathy (described as Jaccoud's arthropathy) may occur.
- **Renal:** disease can range in severity from a benign, focal glomerulitis to a potentially fatal, diffuse membranoproliferative glomerulonephritis.
- **Dermatological:** the butterfly rash over the cheeks is well recognised. It may be photosensitive. Other lesions include discoid lupus, scarring alopecia, Raynaud's disease, livedo reticularis and mucosal (e.g. oral, vaginal) ulcers.
- **Cardiovascular:** hypertension, pericarditis, Libman-Sacks endocarditis.
- **Respiratory:** cough, dyspnoea, pleuritic chest pain and haemoptysis may all occur.
- **Gastrointestinal:** serositis can lead to pain. Impaired motility causes nausea, vomiting and even pseudo-obstruction. Patients may complain of anorexia and weight loss.
- **Neurological:** long-standing headaches and memory problems are common. Patients may have a history of seizures. Occasionally, there may be associated psychosis. There may be problems with the vision associated with retinal vasculitis. The most devastating problem is that of strokes.
- **Haematological:** Coomb's positive haemolysis, leucopoenia, thrombocytopaenia.
- **Systemic:** fever, lethargy, generalised lymphadenopathy, splenomegaly.

For mild disease, treatment should be symptomatic. NSAIDs may be used to treat the joint pain. Aspirin helps to reduce the risk of thrombotic episodes and antimalarials (e.g. hydroxychloroquine) can help with the joint and skin problems. Antimalarials may cause irreversible retinopathy and hence visual acuity should be monitored every 6–12 months. For moderate or severe disease immunosuppression is necessary. Corticosteroids (e.g. prednisolone) should be first line, but long-term maintenance may be achieved with steroid sparing agents such as cyclophosphamide or azathioprine. Cyclosporine, mycophenolate and methotrexate are other alternatives. Some patients are dependent on long-term corticosteroids and these patients should be prescribed adjunct bone protection with, for example, calcium, vitamin D or even bisphosphonates.

Antiphospholipid syndrome

Antiphospholipid syndrome (APS) describes a condition where there is an association between antibodies directed against cell membrane phospholipids and recurrent venous and arterial thrombosis leading to miscarriages, strokes, deep vein thromboses etc. The condition may occur in isolation (Primary APS) or in association with other autoimmune conditions such as SLE (25–50%) (Secondary APS). The pathophysiology of the condition is poorly understood. Treatment in patients with recurrent thrombotic episodes is with anticoagulation. Alternatively prophylaxis can be considered with aspirin and education to eliminate other risk factors (stop smoking and the oral contraceptive pill, treat hypertension and hypercholesterolaemia).

CASE 18: CHANGE IN BOWEL HABIT

Candidate information

You are reviewing patients in the medical outpatient clinic. Your next patient has been referred by his general practitioner with the following letter. Please read the letter and then review the patient.

Dear Doctor,

Re: Mr Donald Corbett

Age: 58 years

Thank you for seeing this man who has been complaining of a change in his bowel habit with diarrhoea for the past few months. I wonder whether he requires a colonoscopy.

Yours sincerely

Subject/Patient's information

Name: Mr Donald Corbett
Age: 58 years
Occupation: Sandwich maker

This gentleman has noticed an increased bowel frequency over the last two months. He had a regular bowel habit, which was once a day, but now goes three or four times each day. There has never been any blood in the motions but he has noticed mucus and slime. Over the past few months he has lost about a half a stone in weight although he was overweight to begin with. His appetite remains normal and there has been no vomiting.

His past medical history includes a history of reactive depression after losing his wife to breast cancer at the age of 42 years. As a child, he broke his left arm after a fall out of a tree. He was diagnosed with diabetes mellitus a few years previously, which has been controlled by diet alone until a few months ago when he was started on metformin.

He takes no other medicines and has no allergies. He doesn't smoke and drinks two pints of beer each evening.

There is no family history of note. He lives alone and has two grown up daughters. For many years now this gentleman has worked in a delicatessen shop making sandwiches, but his bowel habit is of great concern to the owner who has moved him out of the kitchen to the till, which the patient doesn't enjoy and is considering resigning from the job.

Data gathering in the interview

- Greet the patient and introduce yourself.
- Explain to the patient that his GP has referred him with a change in bowel habit and invite him to give you a more detailed account. In particular ask about the frequency and consistency of motions and whether he has noticed any blood or abdominal pain. Go on to ask about systemic symptoms such as lethargy and weight loss.
- Past medical history. Ask about any previous bowel investigations. Make an enquiry on the duration of diabetes and how well it has been controlled over the years and whether he is aware of any damage to any organs as a result of the diabetes. It is worth asking about any previous surgery on the bowels.
- Drug history and allergies. Ask about the medication for his diabetes. Ask how closely the start of the metformin has coincided with the development of the diarrhoea. Specifically ask about any courses of antibiotics (increasing the risk of *Clostridium difficile* infection) the gentleman may have taken and any drugs over the counter. Other drugs that may lead to diarrhoea include NSAIDs, antiarrhythmics (e.g. digoxin) and those containing magnesium. Occasionally patients may develop diarrhoea after they begin eating sweets containing additives such as sorbitol.
- Take the social history. It is particularly important to take a detailed alcohol history and work out whether he has increased the amount drunk. Ask about any recent travel overseas. Enquire about his work and ask if his symptoms are having any impact on his work. Is this leading to stress and a further exacerbation of his symptoms?
- Family history. Is there any history of bowel cancer or inflammatory bowel disease or celiac disease in the family?
- Make the systems enquiry.
- Now confirm that the information is correct and create a problem list and a possible management plan.

Discussion related to the case

According to the British Society of Gastroenterology's Guidelines for the investigation of chronic diarrhoea (*see* BSG website: http://www. bsg.org.uk/) diarrhoea may be defined as the abnormal passage of loose or liquid stools more than three times daily and/or a volume of stool greater than 200 g/day. This definition is useful as patients may present with the problem of diarrhoea when they are simply suffering with loose stools (i.e. reduced consistency without an increase in frequency) or even incontinence.

There is a wide list of differential diagnoses that may explain this man (*see* Table 9). A good clinical history will give great insight into the likely aetiology of this man's symptoms. Perhaps the most important task in a man of this age is to look for clues that may point to the possible diagnosis of cancer. **Cancer** is more likely if the diarrhoea is of recent onset (history shorter than three months) and it is predominantly nocturnal or continuous as opposed to intermittent. Also important is noticeable weight loss and the passage of altered blood. Family history of neoplastic illness (particularly in first-degree relatives) should be actively sought. Family history is also important when **inflammatory bowel disease** (ulcerative colitis and Crohn's disease) is suspected.

Investigations

The investigations are guided by the clinical history. But as a general rule, the following basic investigations should be undertaken in all patients.
- FBC.
- LFT.
- Ca.
- B12, folate and iron studies.
- TFT.
- Celiac serology.
- If an infectious aetiology is suspected, three fresh stool samples should be sent for ova, cysts, parasites and (if appropriate) *Clostridium difficile* toxins.

As a general rule, if the patient is under 45 years of age with typical symptoms (bloating, lower abdominal discomfort, urgency, no bleeding or weight loss) of **functional bowel disease** (e.g. IBS) and the initial investigations are normal, further investigations are not warranted. In patients over 45 years with abnormal initial screening results (e.g. low albumin, anaemia etc) further investigation may be undertaken with flexible sigmoidoscopy plus barium enema to visualise the right side of the colon. Or preferably organise a colonoscopy. Where there is a suspicion of **malabsorption**, the small bowel and the pancreas may need to be investigated. Possible tests include the following.

- **Small bowel:** duodenal biopsies (celiac disease), small bowel follow through (structural abnormality, such as diverticular disease and surgery and secondary to Crohn's disease), jejunal aspirate and culture (for bacterial overgrowth).
- **Pancreas:** imaging, e.g. with CT, MRI/MRCP or ERCP. Functional testing, e.g. faecal elastase.

If there is no obvious cause identified after comprehensive investigations, rare causes should be considered such as bile salt malabsorption (Se-HCAT test), hormone secreting tumours (gut hormone profile measurements) and motility disorders (transit times through the bowels can be measured using various radionucleotide studies which you are not required to know for the purpose of the MRCP exam).

There should always be a high index of suspicion for the possibility of factitious diarrhoea and patients may need to be observed in hospital to objectively quantify stool volume. Stool tests for laxatives may need to be undertaken if abuse is suspected.

Management
Management of patients depends upon the underlying aetiology. But a few basic strategies are outlined here:

- **Bowel cancer:** full 'work up' and assessment to decide the suitability for curative (i.e. resection) or palliative treatment.
- **Functional disease:** reassurance and symptomatic treatments (e.g. antispasmodics, anti-diarrhoeals etc).
- **Inflammatory bowel disease:** aminosalicylates, steroids and immuno-suppressants are the mainstay of management.
- **Celiac disease:** gluten free diet.
- **Pancreatic insufficiency:** pancreatic replacement therapy (e.g. CREON).
- **Small bowel bacterial overgrowth or parasites:** antibiotics.

TABLE 9 Causes of chronic diarrhoea

Colon	• Cancer.
	• Inflammatory bowel disease (ulcerative colitis and Crohn's disease).
Small bowel	• Crohn's disease.
	• Malabsorption enteropathies (celiac disease, Whipple's disease, tropical sprue)
	• Chronic infection, e.g. giardiasis and bacterial overgrowth.
	• Lymphoma.
	• Radiation enteritis.
	• Bile acid malabsorption.
Pancreatic disease	• Cancer.
	• Chronic pancreatitis.
	• Cystic fibrosis (in younger patients).
Non-GI causes	• Endocrine disease: hyperthyroidism, diabetes mellitus, Addison's disease, hypoparathyroidism, hormone secreting tumours.
	• Surgical causes, e.g. small bowel resections.
	• Drugs: there are many including metformin, digoxin, antibiotics, cimetidine, alcohol.
	• Autonomic neuropathy of any cause.
	• Factitious.

Diarrhoea in diabetics

Diabetics are more prone to the development of chronic diarrhoea compared with the normal population. The pathophysiology of the diarrhoea is poorly understood but there are a number of potential causes, which are discussed here.

● Diabetic autonomic neuropathy may lead to abnormalities in small bowel motility and bacterial overgrowth. Excess bacterial deconjugation of bile salts leads to fat malabsorption and steatorrhoea. In addition, excess bile salts irritate the colonic lumen leading to increased secretion and hence.

● Other autoimmune conditions (e.g. thyrotoxicosis, celiac disease) which can cause diarrhoea are particularly associated with Type I diabetes mellitus.

- Oral hypoglycaemic drugs such as sulphonylureas, biguanides (e.g. metformin), acarbose and thiazolidinediones can all lead to diarrhoea, which is often transient and reversible.
- Pancreatic disease leading to diabetes mellitus and pancreatic insufficiency.

CASE 19: TREMOR

Candidate information

You are reviewing patients in the medical outpatient clinic. Your next patient has been referred by his general practitioner with the following letter. Please read the letter and then review the patient.

Dear Doctor,

Re: Mr George Wilkie

Age: 63 years

This gentleman has developed a tremor that is worrying me. I wonder whether he needs treatment for possible Parkinson's disease. He has a history of hypertension and depression, but both of these are well controlled at present. I would very much appreciate your advice.

Yours sincerely

Subject/Patient's information

Name: Mr George Wilkie
Age: 63 years
Occupation: Unemployed

Mr Wilkie first noticed a fine tremor of his hands some weeks ago and sought medical advice. The tremor is present both at rest and on movement. There does not seem to be any problems in initiating movement or with co-ordination and his gait is similarly unaffected. Drinking alcohol does not seem to make any difference to his symptoms. He has, however, noticed that he feels more lethargic than usual and has had bouts of diarrhoea but no vomiting or weight loss. He has previously suffered with severe depression for many years and had attempted suicide at the time of his diagnosis by diverting exhaust fumes to the inside of the car. But fortunately his symptoms have become well controlled since he was started on lithium carbonate some years ago.

Over the past year he has felt so well that he did not even feel it was necessary to go and see his psychiatrist. He is otherwise fit and well except for hypertension that was diagnosed several months ago and his GP started him on furosemide. There are no other medications and he has no known allergies.

He smokes 20 cigarettes each day and drinks alcohol only occasionally. He used to work on a car assembly line but was made redundant over 10 years ago and has not had any regular employment since that time. He lives alone, was never married and has no children. He is one of six children. Three of his siblings and both parents have died of various ailments, the details of which he is uncertain except that one of his brothers successfully committed suicide by jumping off a cliff.

Data gathering in the interview
- Greet the patient and introduce yourself.
- Explain to the patient that his GP has referred him with the 'shakes' and ask him to explain in his own words what the problem is. Ask about the duration of the symptoms and whether there are obvious exacerbating or relieving factors. For example, does drinking alcohol help with the tremor (ensure that the patient understands this term)? Does the tremor worsen with movement or is the same at rest and on movement? Ask whether the tremor is unilateral or bilateral. After ascertaining details of the problem itself, think about potential causes of tremors (such as Parkinson's disease, cerebellar disease, thyrotoxicosis etc) to try to establish an aetiology.
- Past medical history. Ask about any previous medical problems and make note of any illness that may have bearing upon the presenting complaints.
- Drug history and allergies.
- Take the social history. Alcohol, nicotine and caffeine can all be the cause of tremors and hence try to establish the quantity of each consumed on a daily basis. Benign essential tremors often improve with alcohol and it would be well worth establishing such a relationship. Try to establish whether there is a functional impairment associated with the tremor, e.g. is he able to pick up a cup?
- Family history.
- Make the systems enquiry.
- Now confirm that the information is correct and create a problem list and a possible management plan.

Discussion related to the case

A tremor is an involuntary, rhythmic movement usually noticeable in the hands, but may affect other parts of the body such as the head (described as titubation). Most people have a minor tremor, which simply reflects neuromuscular activity used to achieve fine motor control. Stress, anxiety and stimulant drugs such as caffeine may exaggerate this very fine tremor to make it more noticeable.

Also benign in nature is the so-called **essential tremor**. This used to be called a senile tremor as it often presents in older people but now it is well recognised that there is a bimodal age of presentation: The first peak is in early adulthood or adolescence and the second peak is in late adulthood. Women and men are equally affected (although women are more likely to get the tremor of the head) and there may be an inherited component to the condition. Alcohol may temporarily improve symptoms but is not a practical therapy. Alternative pharmacological therapies such as propranolol may prove useful. Occasionally, in extreme circumstances with debilitating tremors, neurosurgical procedures such as a thalamotomy or thalamic stimulation may be considered following consultation at a specialist unit. Essential tremors are most noticeable when the arms are outstretched and often disappear at rest.

Resting tremors do not and suggest more serious pathology, often related to the basal ganglia. Parkinson's disease is a well-recognised cause of such a tremor which is often described as 'pill rolling' as it simulates the action of rolling a pill between the thumb and forefinger. Drugs such as lithium (discussed below) can cause a resting tremor as can Wilson's disease.

When the cerebellum is damaged (e.g. multiple sclerosis, alcoholics, strokes), one of the resultant features is the so-called **intention tremor**. This tremor is most marked at the end of a purposeful movement and the patient may miss their mark when trying to perform at tasks such as pressing a light switch.

The final variety of tremor to be aware of is the **flapping tremor**. The 'flapping' tremor is best demonstrated with the arms stretched out and hands extended. There is a wide variety of causes such as liver failure, hypercapnia, kidney failure, brain damage etc.

Generally speaking, when a patient presents with a tremor, the cause may be identified by the clinical history and examination. Where a structural lesion of the brain is suspected radiological investigations such as CT head or MRI of the brain may be necessary.

Investigations and management

Lithium is commonly used for the treatment of psychiatric conditions such as bipolar disorder and severe depression. It has a relatively narrow therapeutic window and hence toxicity can develop if due caution is not exercised. This includes monitoring of levels and avoiding drugs that may affect the desired level. Diuretics reduce the excretion of lithium and increase the risk of toxicity (loop diuretics are considered safer than thiazides). Mild to moderate **lithium toxicity** results in a fine tremor, lethargy and confusion. Severe toxicity (>2 mmol/L) causes hyper-reflexia, convulsions, cardiac collapse, coma and death.

Patients suspected of lithium toxicity should have the drug stopped immediately and the levels checked. Urea and electrolytes should also be assessed to ascertain the patient's ability to excrete the drug. Moreover, patients with hyponatraemia are at increased risk of developing toxicity. An ECG should be performed to look for evidence of heart block and arrhythmias.

With mild toxicity, observation and adequate hydration should suffice. However, with severe toxicity, renal dialysis may become necessary and management should be carried out in the intensive care unit.

CASE 20: LYMPHADENOPATHY

Candidate information

You are reviewing patients in the medical outpatient clinic. Your next patient has been referred by her general practitioner with the following letter. Please read the letter and then review the patient.

Dear Doctor,

Re: Miss Veronica Smalls

Age: 23 years

I would very much appreciate your advice on the management of this young lady who has been feeling 'run down' and has noticed some weight loss. Examination today showed her to be very thin and worryingly she has enlarged cervical and axillary lymph nodes. I wanted to send her for urgent blood tests but she tells me that she has a needle phobia. We agreed that she would have them done after she had seen you. I am concerned that there may be something seriously wrong with this young lady.

Yours sincerely

Subject/Patient's information

Name: Miss Veronica Smalls
Age: 23 years
Occupation: Unemployed

This lady has been suffering with fatigue for some months, which seems to be progressively worsening. In addition she has noticed significant weight loss (approximately half a stone), which she attributes to diarrhoea (3–4 times/day), which again has been present for several months. There is no steatorrhoea or blood in the stools. Over this period she has also noticed swelling of the 'glands' in her neck, armpits and groin. On occasions there have been fevers and she has had to have several courses of antifungal pastilles to treat oral thrush.

Her past medical history is unremarkable except for a previous, five year long, addiction to heroin. She used to smoke the drug but never injected it as she has a needle phobia. However, to fund the habit she did have to work as a prostitute for two years and often had unprotected sex with different men. She has been drug free for two years now and was actively seeking employment until her symptoms occurred. She is not on any medication at present and has no known allergies.

She lives alone, is not in a relationship and has no pets. On a typical day, she smokes 10 cigarettes but drinks alcohol only very rarely because of her financial worries. There has been no contact with her family for some years, but as far as she is aware there is no serious illness that runs in the family.

Data gathering in the interview

- Greet the patient and introduce yourself.
- Ask her to tell you about her medical problems. Try to quantify the amount of weight lost and the frequency of the diarrhoea. Also ask about any blood in her stools and whether her stools are difficult to flush away, to look for evidence of colitis and pancreatic insufficiency. Ask about the enlarged lymph nodes that are mentioned in the GP's letter and ask questions to explore the possible diagnoses discussed below. Are the lymph nodes increasing in size and are they painful to touch?
- Past medical history. When she tells you about the previous drug habit it is extremely important to ask whether she injected and if so whether she shared needles.
- Drug history and allergies.
- Take the social history. HIV/AIDS is a possible diagnosis and hence her risk for this infection has to be quantified and as such a detailed sexual history must be obtained. Moreover, you should ask about pets to consider the possibility of other infections such as toxoplasmosis, which can cause generalised lymphadenopathy.
- Family history.
- Make the systems enquiry.
- Now confirm that the information is correct and create a problem list and a possible management plan.

Discussion related to the case

Lethargy and weight loss are non-specific symptoms and could be due to a wide variety of clinical conditions. Diarrhoea points to a gastrointestinal disorder but perhaps the most significant feature in this patient is the diffuse lymphadenopathy. The candidate should use this as a handle to generate a differential diagnosis (*see* Table 10). Haematological disease (particularly acute myeloid leukaemia and lymphoma) is possible but perhaps the clinical features and history are most consistent with a diagnosis of HIV infection.

There are four stages of the HIV infection.

- **Stage 1 (Seroconversion).** This is a non-specific viral illness that the patient often undergoes a few weeks after acquiring the infection.
- **Stage 2 (Clinical Latency).** Many months or years may pass with the patient in seemingly good health.
- **Stage 3 (Persistent Generalised Lymphadenopathy).** There are enlarged lymph nodes at two or more sites which persist for longer than three months.
- **Stage 4 (AIDS).** When the CD4 count drops to below $200 \times 10^6/L$ patients develop the so called AIDS defining illnesses. There are many of these and include: Kaposi's sarcoma, mycobacterium avium-intracellulare, pneumocystis, C. pneumonia, oesophageal candidiasis, CMV retinitis, CNS toxoplasmosis etc.

TABLE 10 Causes of generalised lymphadenopathy

Infections	• Bacterial: TB, syphilis, plague, typhoid fever.
	• Viral: HIV, EBV, CMV, rubella, measles, varicella.
	• Fungal: coccidioidomycosis.
	• Protozoal: toxoplasmosis.
Cancers	• Acute leukaemia (AML, ALL).
	• Lymphoma (Hodgkin's and non-Hodgkin's).
Autoimmune disease	• SLE.
	• Juvenile rheumatoid arthritis.
Miscellaneous	• Storage disorders (Gaucher's disease, Niemann-Pick disease).
	• Drug reactions (e.g. phenytoin).
	• Histiocytosis X.

Investigations and management

As a first line, the patient should undergo the following investigations.

- FBC – a low WCC would point to bone marrow failure or HIV infection.
- Peripheral blood film – may show evidence of haematological malignancy.
- U and E – with the ongoing diarrhoea and lethargy it is important to check renal function and to ensure the serum electrolytes are not low.
- HIV test – this should be carried out only after adequate counselling.
- Syphilis serology tests may be considered.
- Chest X-ray – particularly to look for mediastinal lymph node enlargement. A CT scan of the chest may be considered instead.
- Stool microscopy and culture.
- Blood culture as infective endocarditis may rarely present this way.

Perhaps the most important decision is to decide whether a lymph node biopsy should be performed. Generally, it is more important where malignancy is suspected and in this instance it would be reasonable to wait until the results of the initial investigations are back. Management of the patient will depend on the diagnosis. If the patient does turn out to have HIV, she should be referred to a specialist. Generally, a potent combination of ant-iretroviral drugs are initiated when the CD4+ count drops below $<350/\mu L$ and HIV RNA level is greater than 55 000 copies/mL. The treatment is described as highly active anti-retroviral therapy (HAART) and aims to increase the CD4 count and reduce the plasma HIV RNA levels.

CASE 21: HYPERTENSION

Candidate information

You are reviewing patients in the medical outpatient clinic. Your next patient has been referred by her general practitioner with the following letter. Please read the letter and then review the patient.

Dear Doctor,

Re: Mrs Helen Blake

Age: 33 years

I would value your opinion on this rather anxious lady who has been to see me over the past 12 months with a range of ailments. Today she was complaining of a headache, which appears to be very benign in nature and clinically she appeared well but her blood pressure was measured at 192/94. I have commenced a diuretic and will be keeping an eye on her BP but would really value an expert opinion with regards further investigations.

Yours sincerely

Subject/Patient's information

Name: Mrs Helen Blake
Age: 33 years
Occupation: Computer programmer

Over the past 12 months this lady has been greatly troubled by symptoms suggestive of a panic attack. These occur episodically and she typically experiences shortness of breath, palpitations, sweating, light-headedness, 'tingling' fingers, nausea and occasionally vomiting. The attacks last anything from a few seconds to several hours and can be precipitated by various activities such as coughing, sneezing, sexual intercourse and even urination. There were occasions when she felt sure that she was about to die. She has sought advice from her general practitioner on several occasions, only to be told that she was having panic attacks and should try to re-breathe through a paper bag to abort these episodes. On the last occasion, there had been an associated severe headache and on this occasion the doctor had checked her blood pressure, which was found to be markedly elevated. Also worryingly, Mrs Blake has lost over a stone in weight over this period of time.

In the past, she has enjoyed very good health and has never been to see the doctor except to have the oral contraceptive prescribed, which was the only medication she was taking. She has no known allergies, does not smoke or drink alcohol and lives with her husband and four-year-old son. All parents and siblings are all alive and well.

Data gathering in the interview
- Greet the patient and introduce yourself.
- Ask her to tell you about her medical problems. Make a note of her various symptoms and consider possible differential diagnoses. Ask details of the duration of her symptoms and any obvious alleviating or relieving factors. Does she suffer with headaches or visual problems that may be associated with hypertension?
- Past medical history. Has she ever been diagnosed with renal or eye problems? Does she have any other cardiovascular risk factors?
- Drug history and allergies.
- Take the social history. Does she smoke or drink alcohol excessively?
- Family history. See discussion below.
- Make the systems enquiry.
- Now confirm that the information is correct and create a problem list and a possible management plan.

Discussion related to the case
An important clue to the possible diagnosis is the documented hypertension. Possible causes of hypertension are shown in Table 11. The most likely scenario is that this lady is having 'panic attacks' and is incidentally found to have essential hypertension. Or indeed this may be a case of 'white coat' hypertension, particularly if she suffers with anxiety. Another potential cause is the oral contraceptive pill. However, if we choose to examine the history in a purely objective manner, it becomes clear that perhaps the most likely diagnosis is a phaeochromocytoma.

Phaeochromocytomas are rare catecholamine (usually adrenaline or noradrenaline, sometimes dopamine) secreting tumours. In 90% of patients the tumour is benign and confined to the adrenal medulla. Hence a clinical diagnosis may save the life of the patient when it is subsequently confirmed and surgically resected. Morbidity and mortality is usually associated with cardiovascular complications (cardiomyopathy, arrhythmias, ischaemic heart disease and heart failure). Phaeochromocytomas are also associated with rare familial syndromes such as multiple endocrine neoplasia (MEN) 2A and 2B, von Hippel-Lindau syndrome and, of course, neurofibromatosis (von Recklinghausen disease). Hence it is important to consider these conditions when taking the history and to ask for family history of these conditions. The symptoms related to phaeochromocytomas are due to the release of the catecholamines and include 'anxiety', chest pain and palpitations, shortness of breath, nausea, vomiting and weight loss. In fact, it is one of the few causes of weight loss with a normal appetite (others include thyrotoxicosis, malabsorption and diabetes mellitus).

Investigations

These should be carried out by an expert and should include the following.

Blood tests

- FBC – the plasma volume may be constricted, giving rise to a falsely elevated Hb.
- U and E – hypertensive patients should have their renal function tested.
- Glucose – hyperglycaemia or even frank diabetes may be present. The plasma insulin may be inappropriately low.
- Plasma free metadrenalines are up to 99% sensitive for a phaeochromocytoma. These are superior to the catecholamine levels as it is continuously elevated whereas the catecholamines are only elevated during attacks.

Urine tests

- Glycosuria may be present, particularly during attacks.
- 24-hour urine collection for creatinine, total catecholamines, vanillylmandelic acid (VMA), and 4-OH-3-methoxymandelate (HMMA). This is perhaps a useful and readily available first line screening test.

Radiological tests

All patients presenting with hypertension should have a chest X-ray to look for evidence of cardiomyopathy, and heart failure. The 'purists' will also include coarctation of the aorta. In my opinion the chest X-ray findings are not obvious. Tests to be considered for phaeochromocytomas include:

- CT or MRI scanning. MRI is considered to be greatly superior at identifying lesions within the adrenal medulla.
- If a phaeochromocytoma is confirmed biochemically but the imaging with CT/MRI is negative, an MIBG (iodine I 131 – labelled metaiodobenzylguanidine) should be considered. MIBG concentrates within phaeochromocytomas, making them easier to find.
- Positron emission tomography (PET) scanning. Phaeochromocytomas show an increased uptake and hence these studies may be useful but further study is required before it can be considered a routine investigation.

Provocative tests (e.g. with histamine) were carried out in the past but are not recommended now because of their hazardous nature.

Management

Once the diagnosis of a phaeochromocytoma has been established, the treatment of choice is surgical removal. But the operation can be carried out only after hypertension has been controlled to prevent intra-operative hypertensive crisis. The blood pressure can be controlled by a combination of α (e.g. phenoxybenzamine) and β (e.g. propranolol) blockers. The beta-blocker should be initiated only after adequate alpha blockade as unopposed alpha stimulation could in itself precipitate a hypertensive crisis.

The blood pressure should be monitored continuously during the operation, which may be laparoscopic. The anaesthetist needs to be experienced as many anaesthetic drugs could have a detrimental effect during the procedure. Steroids need to be administered if the planned operation is a bilateral adrenalectomy.

TABLE 11 Causes of hypertension

Primary or essential hypertension (approximately 95%).

Secondary hypertension (approximately 5%). Possible causes include the following.

- *Kidney disease:* renal artery stenosis, polycystic kidney disease, chronic pyelonephritis, renal parenchymal disease, urinary tract obstruction, renin-producing tumour, Liddle syndrome.

- *Vascular disease:* coarctation of aorta, vasculitis, collagen vascular disease.

- *Endocrine disease:* oral contraceptives, primary aldosteronism, Cushing syndrome, phaeochromocytoma, congenital adrenal hyperplasia, hyperthyroidism and hypothyroidism, hypercalcaemia, hyperparathyroidism, acromegaly.

- *Neurological disease:* brain tumour, intracranial hypertension, bulbar poliomyelitis.

- *Miscellaneous conditions:* pregnancy related (e.g. pre-eclampsia), drugs and toxins (cyclosporine, erythropoietin, alcohol, cocaine, adrenergic medications).

CASE 22: ABDOMINAL PAIN

Candidate information

You are reviewing patients in the medical outpatient clinic. Your next patient has been referred by his general practitioner with the following letter. Please read the letter and then review the patient.

Dear Doctor,

Re: Mr Paul Sweeney

Age: 58 years

Many thanks for your expert opinion on this chap who has been complaining of abdominal pain and has lost half a stone in weight. I am concerned that I may be missing a serious problem and wonder whether he needs a gastroscopy. Recent blood tests, including a FBC, U and E and LFTs, were normal. Serum glucose and lipids were elevated but he is a known diabetic and is on cholesterol lowering medication.

Yours sincerely

Subject/Patient's information

Name: Mr Paul Sweeney
Age: 58 years
Occupation: Garage owner

For some months this gentleman has been suffering with abdominal pain, mainly confined to the epigastric region. The pain typically comes on a few hours after eating and at times can be severe. Now the pain bothers him so much that he is actually frightened to eat. As a consequence there has been weight loss of approximately half a stone (around 3 kg). There is never any nausea or vomiting and his bowel habit is normal. The stools are of normal colour and consistency and flush easily.

Three years ago Mr Sweeney suffered an acute myocardial infarct after a lengthy history of angina. At the time he underwent coronary angioplasty and was advised to stop smoking, which he did for six months then restarted and is now smoking 20 cigarettes a day. He knows it's bad for him but feels that it is his only pleasure in life, particularly as he has had to stop drinking beer because of his abdominal pains. He used to drink four pints of lager every night. He is known to suffer with diabetes, has a high blood pressure and is waiting to see a specialist for pains in his calves. His current medication consists of gliclazide, atorvastatin and ramipril. There are no allergies.

He owns his own car workshop and is financially secure. Lives with his wife and has four children who have all moved out. His parents died many years ago: father aged 62 years of a heart attack and mother 76 years following a long battle with bowel cancer.

Data gathering in the interview

- Greet the patient and introduce yourself.
- Tell the patient that his doctor has referred him because of his abdominal pain and ask him to tell you more about his symptoms. Enquire into the character of the pain (colicky? continuous?), the site, duration and any obvious exacerbating or relieving factors. Also find out how the pain is related to meals and whether there has been any weight loss. Check to see if there has been any nausea or vomiting or any change in bowel habit. Are there any features of pancreatic disease? In view of the weight loss enquire into the possibility of dysphagia.
- Past medical history. Look for evidence of vascular disease in the past medical history. Ask if he has ever had any abdominal operations, which may give rise to intra-abdominal adhesions or you can practically exclude gallstone colic if he has previously had a cholecystectomy. Is there a history of pancreatic disease or peptic ulcer disease and has he ever had a gastroscopy?
- Drug history and allergies. Is he taking aspirin or NSAIDs, which may precipitate ulcers?
- Take the social history. It is particularly important to take a detailed smoking and alcohol history because of their connections to conditions leading to chronic abdominal pain (e.g. peptic ulcer disease, gastro-oesophageal reflux disease, chronic pancreatitis, hepatitis). Ask about potential exposure to lead (although this is less likely in the UK these days) and consider the possibility of intestinal infestation with parasites by asking about foreign travel.

- Family history. It is very important to ask about family history of Crohn's disease and upper gastrointestinal cancer.
- Make the systems enquiry.
- Now confirm that the information is correct and create a problem list and a possible management plan.

Discussion related to the case

There is no doubt that this man has multiple risk factors for atherosclerosis (smoker, diabetes mellitus, hyperlipidaemia and family history) and has a past medical history of ischaemic heart disease and possible peripheral vascular disease. This fact and the clinical history make the diagnosis of chronic mesenteric ischaemia very attractive. However, this is a relatively rare diagnosis and all other potential causes of his pain should be considered. These include: peptic ulcer disease, chronic pancreatitis, cholecystitis, Crohn's disease, intestinal TB, lymphoma, parasitic infestation, chronic lead poisoning and porphyria. Clearly some of these are much more common than others, depending on which part of the world you are in. The medical history clearly plays an extremely important role in directing the doctor to the likely diagnosis. For instance, unlike this case, pain improves with eating in patients with peptic ulcer disease.

Investigations and management

In view of this man's age and history of weight loss it is absolutely mandatory to proceed to an urgent gastroscopy (*see* NICE guidelines on dyspepsia). Other tests worth considering are the following.

- Repeat of the blood tests and include inflammatory markers (CRP, ESR) to look for evidence of active inflammation.
- ECG to ensure this is not referred cardiac pain!
- An abdominal ultrasound scan to explore the possibility of gall-stones and to visualise the pancreas. Often the ultrasound scan gives poor views of the pancreas and a CT scan may be more favourable. A mesenteric duplex ultrasound scan is a non-invasive method of analysing flow through the vessels.
- Small bowel follow through to explore the possibility of small bowel disease, e.g. Crohn's disease, lymphoma or intestinal TB.
- If there is a strong clinical suspicion that this is mesenteric ischaemia and other tests are negative, a mesenteric angiogram may be undertaken.

Once mesenteric ischaemia is established, the patient can be commenced on anticoagulation with warfarin to reduce the risk of acute infarction and, if deemed medically fit (advice from a cardiologist may be necessary at this point), surgery should be considered. Surgical intervention includes endarterectomy and bypass procedures. Stenting is being evaluated.

CASE 23: BLUE FINGERS

Candidate information

You are reviewing patients in the medical outpatient clinic. Your next patient has been referred by her general practitioner with the following letter. Please read the letter and then review the patient.

Dear Doctor,

Re: Mrs Bianca Sawyer

Age: 27 years

I would really value your opinion on this young woman who came in to the clinic for a routine health check and was found to be cyanosed. I am concerned that I am missing a medical problem here and wonder whether she warrants further investigation.

Yours sincerely

Subject/Patient's information

Name: Mrs Bianca Sawyer
Age: 27 years
Occupation: Cinema cashier

This lady was invited to her doctor's surgery for a routine health check. While there, it was noted that her fingers were blue, which concerned the doctor and prompted today's referral. Mrs Sawyer had not been concerned about this, as she had noticed the discoloration in her fingers for many months, perhaps even a few years. The fingers usually turned blue or pale white, often with cold or anxiety. But subsequently the colour returned to normal or they became very red. There had been no other associated problems of any description and she has previously been fit and well.

As a child she was troubled with asthma and had to have her appendix removed after developing acute abdominal pain. The only medication she takes is the oral contraceptive pill. She is allergic to latex, which can cause her to develop wheezing, but has no drug allergies as far as she is aware. She smokes 10 cigarettes a day and drinks about two bottles of wine each week. Her sister suffers with schizophrenia and her mother died of pneumonia, but her father and two brothers are alive and well.

Data gathering in the interview

- Greet the patient and introduce yourself.
- Tell her that her doctor has referred her because she was noticed to have blue fingers. Ask her to tell you more about this problem. It is important to get very specific details about any changes in colour, the duration of the symptoms and any associated problems.
- Past medical history. Specifically ask about any history of musculo-skeletal problems. Is there a history of migraines?
- Drug history and allergies. Particularly ask about the oral contraceptive pill.
- Take the social history. Smoking history is crucial. It would be worth taking a brief occupational history, particularly to check for exposure to vibrating tools and lead or PVC. (These are unlikely causes of her cyanosis, but shows that you are thinking. Arsenic is much less likely and I wouldn't bother asking about it.)
- Family history.
- Make the systems enquiry.
- Now confirm that the information is correct and create a problem list and a possible management plan.

Discussion related to the case

This lady's symptoms are highly suggestive of **Raynaud's disease**. This should be distinguished from **Raynaud's phenomenon**, where there are similar clinical changes but the condition is associated with a number of clinical conditions (*see* Table 12). The condition affects the peripheral body parts, usually the hands, and is characterised by vasospasm leading to distinct colour changes. Initially there is pallor (white) and/or cyanosis (blue) followed by a hyperaemic phase leading to erythema (red). With advanced and severe cases, tissue necrosis may occur. There may be associated numbness or pain.

Investigations and management

Often the clinical history is conclusive of a primary Raynaud's disease and no further investigation needs to be undertaken. However, if there is a clinical suspicion that this may be Raynaud's phenomenon secondary to one of the conditions outlined in Table 12, the appropriate investigations should be undertaken.

Management consists of general measures such as patient education (avoid triggering factors such as the cold and stop smoking.). Strategies for active re-warming may be considered, e.g. heated gloves. There is some data to support the use of calcium channel blockers and ACE inhibitors but there is no proven role for anti-platelet agents or anti-coagulation. The role of sympathectomy (either cervical or digital) is controversial but may be useful in some patients.

Clearly if patients are suffering with Raynaud's phenomenon, then the underlying condition needs to be addressed and treated.

TABLE 12 Conditions associated with Raynaud's phenomenon

Autoimmune disease	• scleroderma, rheumatoid arthritis, SLE, dermatomyositis, vasculitis and Sjögren's syndrome.
Cancers	• leukaemia, myeloma, lymphoma, lung cancer and others.
Environmental factors	• vibration injury, lead poisoning, PVC exposure, frostbite, arsenic exposure.
Infections	• hepatitis B and C (especially associated with mixed or type 3 cryoglobulinemia), *Mycoplasma* infections (with cold agglutinins).
Haematological conditions	• paroxysmal nocturnal hemoglobinuria, polycythaemia, Waldenström macroglobulinemia, monoclonal cryoglobulinemia.
Primary pulmonary hypertension	
Drugs	• oral contraceptives, ergot alkaloids, bromocriptine, beta-adrenergic blocking drugs, antineoplastics (e.g. vinca alkaloids, bleomycin, cisplatin), cyclosporine, alfa-interferon.
Metabolic	• diabetes mellitus, acromegaly, myxoedema, phaeochromocytoma.

CASE 24: HYPOKALAEMIA

Candidate information

You are reviewing patients in the medical outpatient clinic. Your next patient has been referred by her general practitioner with the following letter. Please read the letter and then review the patient.

Dear Doctor,

Re: Miss Wendy Probert

Age: 33 years

This young lady has been complaining of lethargy for some time. To investigate potential causes she had some blood tests done which showed a potassium value of 3.1 mM/L. I wonder whether this is causing her symptoms and would greatly value your advice regarding further management. She has a history of hypertension and has seen the practice nurse for dietary advice regarding her obesity, but is otherwise fit and well.

Yours sincerely

Subject/Patient's information

Name: Miss Wendy Probert
Age: 33 years
Occupation: Shop assistant

This lady went to see her GP, as she had been feeling lethargic and generally 'run down' for some weeks. One of the blood tests was abnormal which prompted the referral to this clinic today. There have been no other symptoms.

She was diagnosed with hypertension three years previously, for which she takes bendrofluazide 2.5 mg od and ramipril 5 mg od. In addition she has the tendency to suffer with constipation and takes lactulose, as required. Miss Probert is very self-conscious about her weight. She has been 'yo-yo' dieting for the whole of her adult life and as a child was bullied because of her obesity. A friend had told her that laxatives can encourage weight loss and over the last couple of months she has been taking an extra lactulose dose and Sennakot tablets which she buys over the counter. She uses the laxatives secretly, but will volunteer the information if directly questioned by the doctor at the interview today. There are no known allergies, she doesn't smoke and drinks only occasionally. She lives alone, but her parents live close by and are fit and well.

Data gathering in the interview
- Greet the patient and introduce yourself.
- Ask the patient to tell you about her medical problems. Take details of how long she has been suffering with lethargy and ask about other symptoms that can be associated with hypokalaemia such as nausea/ vomiting, palpitations, paraesthesia etc. Considering common causes of hypokalaemia (see discussion below), ask about any history of diarrhoea and vomiting. It would be pertinent to ask about medication that may have caused the hypokalaemia and specifically ask her whether she is on diuretics (or water tablets) and laxatives.
- Past medical history. See discussion for conditions that may lead to hypokalaemia.
- Drug history and allergies. As above.
- Take the social history.
- Family history.
- Make the systems enquiry.
- Now confirm that the information is correct and create a problem list and a possible management plan.

Discussion related to the case
Hypokalaemia is a common medical problem and can be caused by a wide range of conditions (*see* Table 13). Common causes include gastrointestinal loss (diarrhoea and vomiting) and the use of thiazide or loop diuretics. This lady clearly has both of these risk factors and is at risk of developing hypokalaemia. This case illustrates the importance of teasing out relevant information from the patient who doesn't otherwise volunteer this readily, for a range of reasons (probably embarrassment in this instance).

Investigations and management

It is best to adopt a commonsense approach to this patient when organising investigations. As suggested above the likely aetiology for her symptoms is GI loss and diuretics. An appropriate strategy would be to simply stop the diuretics and laxatives and monitor the serum potassium. As she is symptomatic a short course of oral potassium supplements may be appropriate. Intravenous supplements are only necessary when patients are found to have severe hypokalaemia (below 2.6 mM/L).

Because of the history of hypertension, the possibility of hyperaldosteronism and perhaps Cushing's syndrome should be considered as possible causes of the hypokalaemia. If the above strategy fails to resolve the problem then appropriate investigations for these conditions should be organised. In addition an atrial blood gas analysis (to look for alkalosis), an ECG (with characteristic changes of flat T waves and U waves) and serum magnesium levels should be organised and reviewed.

TABLE 13 Causes of hypokalaemia

GI loss	• diarrhoea (including laxative and enema use), vomiting, ileal loop.
Medication effects	• diuretics, laxatives, steroids, beta-adrenergic agonists, aminoglycosides, theophylline, insulin.
Renal losses	• hyperaldosteronism, renal tubular acidosis, magnesium depletion (e.g. in alcoholics), genetic conditions (e.g. Bartter's syndrome, Gitelman's syndrome).
Others	• alkalosis, malnutrition, parenteral nutrition.

CASE 25: ABDOMINAL AND LEG SWELLING

Candidate information

You are reviewing patients in the medical outpatient clinic. Your next patient has been referred by his general practitioner with the following letter. Please read the letter and then review the patient.

Dear Doctor,

Re: Mr Eric MacKay

Age: 44 years

I would very much appreciate your expert opinion on this nice man who has developed swelling of his abdomen and legs, confirmed on clinical examination. He has enjoyed good health previously except for a diagnosis of epilepsy, for which he is on medication.

Yours sincerely

Subject/Patient's information

Name: Mr Eric MacKay
Age: 44 years
Occupation: Teacher

This man has been referred for a specialist opinion regarding his abdominal and leg swelling which he has noticed over the last few weeks. The problem has been progressive and first came to attention when he found it difficult to fit into any of his trousers. He also feels continuously tired and listless and often suffers with bouts of nausea and vomiting. Some mornings there has been a noticeable yellow tinge to the whites of the eyes, but no change in the colour of the urine or stools.

One year previously, Mr MacKay had suffered a fit at the school where he had been teaching and was rushed to hospital. The following morning the doctor on duty had confidently diagnosed epilepsy and started him on phenytoin tablets before discharge. The past medical history is otherwise unremarkable. There are no known drug allergies.

He is a non-smoker but drinks heavily. Mr MacKay has always enjoyed a drink, and would have a few beers most nights of the week. However, he had started drinking very heavily about 18 months ago after the breakdown of his marriage. He subsequently lost his driving licence and a few months ago was suspended from work. Now he is drinking 3–4 litres of cider each day, which often starts first thing in the morning. His mother is alive and well but his father died aged 74 years, of lung cancer. One of his brothers died of liver failure, thought to be related to alcohol abuse, at the age of 38 years.

Data gathering in the interview

- Greet the patient and introduce yourself.
- Ask him to tell you about his abdominal and leg swelling. Particularly ask about the duration of symptoms and the rate of progression, if any. Ask about any related symptoms. The abdominal swelling is likely to be ascites hence explore the possibility of underlying liver disease. Has he noticed any jaundice or easy bruising?
- Past medical history. Find out the exact nature of the fit and whether there had been any further episodes. Try to establish whether the diagnosis of epilepsy is a secure one. Has he previously been diagnosed with liver disease?
- Drug history and allergies. Is he on diuretics?
- Take the social history. For obvious reasons it is extremely important to take a very detailed history of alcohol consumption (see below). Also look for other potential risk factors for developing liver disease such as tattoos, blood transfusions etc.
- Family history. Alcoholism can run in families.
- Make the systems enquiry.
- Now confirm that the information is correct and create a problem list and a possible management plan.

Discussion related to the case

Alcohol is perhaps the favourite drug of the Western world. According to the Department of Health, its misuse costs the NHS an estimated £1.6 billion each year (the cost to society in terms of health, crime and loss of productivity is estimated at £20 billion each year). Each year there are 150,000 hospital episodes with 22,000 deaths related to alcohol in the UK. Moreover, 35% of all A&E attendances involve alcohol. For these reasons, it is essential that all doctors recognise alcohol abuse early so that patients may be referred for appropriate counselling or treatment.

Assessing an individual's alcohol intake can be difficult for two reasons: It is difficult to standardise alcohol consumption and patients can often be very guarded or even deceitful when reporting their consumption. Often people underestimate the amount of alcohol they consume. When taking the history, specifically ask about the type of beverage (beer, wine, spirit etc), its alcohol content (common beers can be anything from 2–10% in alcohol), and the size of glass used. From the information obtained, try to establish the number of units being consumed each week. Some people are binge drinkers. They may go for weeks without a drink and then drink 20 units in one sitting.

There are numerous screening tools to identify alcohol misuse. The gold standard was developed by the World Health Organization and is known as the Alcohol Use Disorder Identification Test (AUDIT). However, this is quite cumbersome and not practical for the setting of the MRCP PACES exam. Briefer versions such as the AUDIT-PC and the FAST have been developed and indeed there is even the one question version. The Single Alcohol Screening Questionnaire (SASQ) involves asking the patient, 'When was the last time you had six (women)/eight (men) units of alcohol on any one occasion? A positive result is denoted by an answer within the last three months and the patient should be given appropriate advice (*see* www.alcoholconcern.org.uk). Perhaps the most useful and commonly used tool is the CAGE questionnaire:

- Have you ever felt you should cut down on your drinking?
- Have people annoyed you by criticising your drinking?
- Have you ever felt guilty about your drinking?
- Have you ever had a drink first thing in the morning to get rid of a hangover (an eye opener)?

Investigations
This man is likely to have advanced liver disease as a result of his drinking and warrants further investigations. The liver is a highly complex organ and no single test can assess overall hepatic function.

Blood tests
- **LFT, albumin and GGT.** Bilirubin will rise if there is cholestasis either due to obstruction or hepatocellular necrosis/inflammation. The liver enzymes (AST and ALT) are both exquisitely sensitive indicators of

hepatocellular injury. ALP is a bile canalicular enzyme that is dispro-portionately increased in cholestasis. GGT is a microsomal enzyme that is also easily inducible, for example by alcohol, and hence is often elevated in alcoholics. Albumin is synthesised by the liver and hence low values suggest reduced hepatic synthetic function implying advanced liver disease.

- **INR/PT.** The liver also synthesises vitamin K dependent clotting factors. So increasing INR/PT values also imply reduced synthetic function.
- **FBC.** Likely to show macrocytosis and thrombocytopaenia.

These tests should be performed routinely. The likely aetiology for this man's liver disease is alcohol. However, alcohol abuse can unmask other underlying conditions and hence it is useful to carry out blood tests to exclude other potential causes of liver disease. These include serum ferritin, hepatitis B and C serology and immunological tests (AMA, ANA, SMA, LKM and immunoglobulins). Patients with established cirrhosis are at a greatly increased risk of developing hepatomas of the liver and alpha-fetoprotein provides a useful screening test.

Radiological test
Ultrasonography is readily available and widely used and can give very useful information regarding the presence of focal lesions and detection of fatty liver (steatosis), which results in a diffuse increase in echogenicity. Moreover, Doppler studies can help to establish the patency of hepatic vessels, such as the hepatic and portal veins. CT scans may give little additional information and indeed are inferior to ultrasonography in terms of visualising the biliary tract.

Liver biopsy
This is a simple procedure but is only carried out occasionally because of possible complications (bleeding, pain, infection). But it is useful in terms of staging of the liver disease.

Management
Management needs to be tailored to each individual patient but general measures include the following.
- Advice and support to encourage alcohol abstinence.
- Nutritional advice and supplements (including vitamins) where necessary.

- Diuretics to treat ascites and oedema.
- Screen for and treat oesophageal varices.
- Treat complications such as encephalopathy, subacute bacterial peritonitis.

CASE 26: PRURITIS

Candidate information

You are reviewing patients in the medical outpatient clinic. Your next patient has been referred by her general practitioner with the following letter. Please read the letter and then review the patient.

Dear Doctor,

Re: Mrs Sandra Billington

Age: 59 years

Thank you for your advice on this lady who has been suffering with pruritis for some months. I have tried calamine lotion and antihistamines with no benefit. I am at my wit's end and frankly do not know what else I can offer her.

Yours sincerely

Subject/Patient's information

Name: Mrs Sandra Billington
Age: 59 years
Occupation: Switchboard operator

This lady has been suffering with a generalised pruritis (itching) for some weeks. Her GP tried some calamine lotion and antihistamine tablets, but these made very little difference to her symptoms and hence she has been referred to this clinic for further advice. She has also noted a non-specific pain in her chest associated with mild breathlessness and half a stone (approximately 3 kg) weight loss. On occasions, this lady has been troubled with terrible sweats. These sweats are worse at night and on occasions she has had to get up and change her clothes. There is no noticeable jaundice.

In the past she has suffered with severe depression in her mid-thirties, and made a suicide attempt. This is well controlled now. She also has a history of hypothyroidism and at the age of 48 years a lump was removed from her left breast, which was found to have a malignant focus. The surgeon who carried out the procedure has since discharged her. Her medications consist of imipramine, thyroxine and *Ginkgo biloba* (which she buys over the counter). She may be allergic to penicillin, because she developed a mild rash on ingestion.

She stopped smoking six years ago and never drinks alcohol. She lives with her husband and two daughters. She normally works as a switchboard operator in the hospital, but has had to take time off work because of her symptoms. There is no significant family history.

Data gathering in the interview
- Greet the patient and introduce yourself.
- Tell the patient that her GP has referred her because of her itching and invite her to tell you more about this problem. Ask whether the itching is localised to certain parts of the body or generalised. Ask about changes to the skin (rash, lichenification, excoriations).
- Past medical history. Explore the possibility of this lady suffering from any of the conditions discussed below, known to cause generalised pruritis. Specifically ask her if she has noticed any jaundice. Has she had night sweats? Has she noticed enlarged glands?
- Drug history and allergies. Certain drugs, such as opiates, may cause pruritis.
- Take the social history. What impact are her symptoms having on her work and might they be attributable to her vocation?
- Family history.
- Make the systems enquiry.
- Now confirm that the information is correct and create a problem list and a possible management plan.

Discussion related to the case
A generalised pruritis may be due to a skin condition or systemic illness (Table 14). A relatively common cause of pruritis in middle-aged women is primary biliary cirrhosis. This lady has no features to suggest this condition but she does have obvious features of Hodgkin's disease and should be investigated aggressively.

Investigations and management
This lady should have urgent **blood tests** requested which should include:

- FBC – polycythaemia and bone marrow involvement
- UE – renal failure
- LFT – liver disease
- LDH – may be elevated in Hodgkin's disease
- TFT – to look for thyroid disease.

A chest X-ray is mandatory. If it confirms the presence of mediastinal lymph nodes a CT guided biopsy may be appropriate.

The management depends on the confirmation of underlying condition, which in this case is likely to be Hodgkin's disease.

TABLE 14 Causes of generalised pruritis

Skin conditions	• Dry skin and sunburn. • Dermatitis of any cause. • Psoriasis. • Urticaria. • Scabies and lice. • Lichen planus.
Systemic illness	• Chronic renal failure. • Cholestasis, e.g. secondary to primary biliary cirrhosis. • Haematological disease: polycythaemia, Hodgkin's disease, iron deficiency. • Endocrine: diabetes mellitus, thyroid disease, hypoparathyroidism. • Others: drugs (e.g. opioids), neuropathic pruritis, delusional.

CASE 27: POLYDIPSIA AND POLYURIA

Candidate information

You are reviewing patients in the medical admissions unit. Your next patient has been referred by her general practitioner with the following letter. Please read the letter and then review the patient.

Dear Doctor,

Re: Mrs Jennifer Hardcastle

Age: 48 years

Please advise on the management of this lady who has been complaining of an insatiable thirst and frequent urination. I have checked her bloods and her serum calcium, fasting glucose, renal and liver biochemistry as well as a full blood count were all entirely normal. She has also had a glucose tolerance test on two occasions, both of which were negative for diabetes mellitus. ECG today showed mild ST depression, but she does have a history of angina. I am uncertain about further investigations and would value your opinion. Thank you.

Yours sincerely

Subject/Patient's information

Name: Mrs Jennifer Hardcastle
Age: 48 years
Occupation: Unemployed

This lady has been referred by her GP because of her constant thirst and frequent urination. This problem has been progressively worsening over the last month. It is not unusual for her to drink 15 litres of water (she has been measuring it) and pass urine over 20 times in a 24-hour period. This includes several trips to the bathroom during the course of the night. There has been no noticeable weight loss and her appetite is normal (despite feeling nauseous and suffering with intermittent diarrhoea) but she does feel lethargic and generally tired.

She is known to have suffered with schizophrenia since the age of 19 years. Ten years ago she was involved in a road traffic accident where she sustained significant head injury and a spinal fracture, which required a prolonged hospital admission. Three years ago she underwent a hysterectomy for menorrhagia. In addition she is known to suffer with angina. Her current medication consists of GTN spray used on a prn basis, isosorbide mononitrate, atenolol, aspirin, perindopril and lithium. She has also been taking ibuprofen for back pain over the past month. There are no known allergies. She used to be under the care of a psychiatrist, who retired two years ago. She was supposed to be followed up by another psychiatrist but has not received an appointment and as she has been symptom free has not bothered to chase up the appointment.

She smokes heavily and drinks beer occasionally and lives with her husband. There are no children. There is no significant family history.

Data gathering in the interview

- Greet the patient and introduce yourself.
- Invite the patient to tell you about her medical problems. Try to quantify the amount of water she is drinking and the frequency of urination. It is important to ask about nocturia as patients with psychogenic polydipsia tend not get up in the night to pass urine.
- Past medical history. Is she known to suffer with diabetes mellitus or renal impairment? Does she have a history of psychiatric illness, which may necessitate the use of lithium therapy?
- Drug history and allergies. Ask about her dose of lithium and find out whether the levels are monitored. Is she on calcium supplements?
- Take the social history.
- Family history.
- Make the systems enquiry.
- Now confirm that the information is correct and create a problem list and a possible management plan.

Discussion related to the case

Table 15 shows possible causes of polydipsia and polyuria. The most likely cause for this lady's symptoms (in view of the GP's investigations) is nephrogenic diabetes insipidus secondary to lithium toxicity. Cranial diabetes insipidus is a less likely possibility as is psychogenic polydipsia (particularly as she is getting symptoms of nocturia).

Investigations and management

- Biochemistry including Ca may be repeated.
- Serum lithium levels should be checked as a priority.
- ECG can be repeated. ST depression and T wave inversion are frequently associated with lithium toxicity.
- A simultaneous measurement of serum and urine osmolality. If there is any doubt about the cause of the symptoms, a water deprivation test may be carried out (see below).

TABLE 15 Causes of polydipsia and polyuria

Cranial diabetes insipidus

- Primary.
- Acquired (injury, hypophysectomy, suprasellar and intrasellar).
- tumours, infections (encephalitis or meningitis), histiocytosis, granulomas.
- (sarcoidosis or TB) and vascular lesions (e.g. aneurysm).

Nephrogenic diabetes insipidus

- Congenital.
- Acquired (chronic renal disease, drugs (lithium, demeclocycline), Systemic.
- disease (myeloma, sickle cell disease) Hypercalcaemia.

Psychogenic polydipsia

Osmotic diuresis, e.g. glucose (diabetes mellitus).

Water deprivation test

This test must be carried out under supervision as patient may become severely dehydrated. Also, the patient can be monitored for surreptitious water consumption. The patient's water intake is withheld. Baseline and hourly measurements of urine osmolality and body weight are taken until the weight drops by more than 3%. At this point sc vasopressin is administered and final measurements are taken an hour later. In healthy individuals the test leads to a urine osmolality 2–4 times greater than plasma osmolality. Administration of vasopressin results in less than 9% increment in urine osmolality. In complete central DI, urine remains dilute despite concentrated serum. However, the urine responds to and becomes concentrated after vasopressin administration. There is no such response to vasopressin in patients with nephrogenic DI.

If this patient is found to be lithium toxic, management consists of withholding the drug. In severe cases haemodialysis may be necessary. Often the diabetes insipidus is reversible upon cessation of the lithium.

CASE 28: DIPLOPIA

Candidate information

You are reviewing patients in the medical outpatient clinic. Your next patient has been referred by her general practitioner with the following letter. Please read the letter and then review the patient.

Dear Doctor,

Re: Miss Wendy Askwith

Age: 29 years

I am concerned about this lady who came to the surgery complaining of 'double vision'. Clinical examination was unremarkable except for nystagmus upon lateral gaze. There was no evidence of a ptosis. But I remain concerned as she's never been to the surgery previously and strikes me as a sensible person.

Yours sincerely

Subject/Patient's information

Name: Miss Wendy Askwith
Age: 29 years
Occupation: Librarian

This lady has been concerned about her vision for some weeks. Initially she noticed pain in her right eye, which caused her vision to become blurred. She had organised an appointment with the optician, but became very concerned when over the weekend she had developed distinct double vision. The two images are adjacent to one another (horizontal images) and there is only a single image when she covers one of the eyes. She has also noticed numbness and tingling in her arms and feels generally fatigued.

In the past she has been in hospital only once as a teenager when she developed meningitis. But she made a full recovery.

She does not take any medication and has no allergies. She has never smoked cigarettes and drinks alcohol only at weekends and has never used illicit drugs. She is an only child and lives with her parents. Her mother suffers with severe rheumatoid arthritis. Because of her visual problems, she has been off work and is worried that she will not be able to return to work until the problem resolves.

Data gathering in the interview

- Greet the patient and introduce yourself.
- Invite the patient to tell you about her medical problems. Clarify whether the diplopia is horizontal, vertical or oblique and whether it corrects on covering one eye. Has she noticed any pain in the eye (e.g. due to optic neuritis), or loss of visual acuity? Are there any associated neurological symptoms (e.g. tremor, unsteadiness, reduced co-ordination)?
- Past medical history. Specifically ask about diabetes mellitus.
- Drug history and allergies.
- Take the social history. What work does she do and are the symptoms going to compromise her ability to function?
- Family history.
- Make the systems enquiry.
- Now confirm that the information is correct and create a problem list and a possible management plan.

Discussion related to the case

This lady's profile (female, Caucasian and around 30 years) and symptoms are strongly suggestive of a diagnosis of multiple sclerosis. This is an idiopathic demyelinating disease, which tends to be progressive. But often there is a relapsing/remitting pattern. Often, in the early years, there is full recovery between episodes but over time the patient becomes progressively disabled. The degree of disability is difficult to predict and some patients may remain very active for decades.

Investigations

No test is pathognomonic, but each helps to confirm the diagnosis. Tests to be considered should include the following.

- CSF analysis. Elevated protein and selective increase in immuno-globulin G (e.g. oligoclonal bands, free kappa chains).
- Delayed visual, auditory and somatosensory evoked potentials.

- MRI is more sensitive compared to CT in detecting plaques.

Management

Management is generally supportive as there is no cure for the condition. Treatments include the following.

- Baclofen for spasticity.
- Antidepressants if the patient develops clinical depression.
- Bladder catheterisation if there is bladder dysfunction.
- Laxatives.
- Men may require impotence treatment.

There is good evidence that certain treatments may shorten relapses. These include IV methylprednisolone, B Interferon 1b and plasmapheresis.

CASE 29: BACKACHE

Candidate information

You are reviewing patients in the medical outpatient clinic. Your next patient has been referred by his general practitioner with the following letter. Please read the letter and then review the patient.

Dear Doctor,

Re: Mr Giles Francis

Age: 31 years

I would very much appreciate your opinion on this young man who is complaining of a back pain. I am worried that this may be secondary to renal problems. However, blood tests including a full blood count, urea and electrolytes are all normal. I wonder whether he needs an ultrasound examination of his renal tract.

Yours sincerely

Subject/Patient's information

Name: Mr Giles Francis
Age: 31 years
Occupation: Butcher

This gentleman has been suffering with a backache for some months. It is affecting his lower back, radiating to his buttocks. The pain tends to be worse at night and on occasions has woken him from sleep. He had suffered with a similar episode in the previous year but not as severe and the pain had eventually resolved. This time, simple analgesics such as aspirin and paracetamol had initially proved useful but now are not controlling the symptoms. However, ibuprofen does ease the pain. In addition to the pain, he is also suffering with stiffness, which is worse first thing in the morning but tends to ease during the course of the day. Additionally, he is finding his spinal mobility to be greatly reduced. It is very difficult to turn from side to side or indeed to stand up straight.

These symptoms are interfering with Mr Francis' ability to work as a butcher as it involves lifting heavy joints of meat and has had to take time off. There has also been a problem with pain in his right eye, which have become quite red on occasions. He has not noticed any problem on passing urine. There have been no fevers, night sweats or weight loss. Bowel habit has always been regular, opening once daily.

There is no history of serious illness and he does not take any other medication. He is allergic to latex, which causes a rash.

Mr Francis has been married for 10 years to his childhood sweatheart and he has never had any other sexual relationships. He smokes 10 cigarettes per day and drinks 20 units of beer each week. There is no family history of note.

Data gathering in the interview

- Greet the patient and introduce yourself.
- Invite the patient to tell you about his medical problems. Ask about the duration of the pain symptoms and whether there are obvious exacerbating factors such as movement. Are there any features to suggest sciatica? (Shooting pain down the buttock and leg, often exacerbated by coughing and straining, which suggests disc herniation). Back pain due to infection or cancer does not improve with lying down flat and it is very important to clarify whether the pain improves at night. Also ask about morning stiffness. Are there features of cord compression? (Ask about bowel and bladder dysfunction and neurological signs in the lower limbs.) Ask about systemic symptoms such as fever and weight loss.
- Past medical history. As the GP has raised the possibility of renal disease, ask the patient if he has had any kidney problems and whether he has noticed any dysuria or haematuria. The history of dysuria and urethral discharge may be elicited at this point; alternatively it may only be raised later in the systemic enquiry. Is there a history of back problems or spinal operations? Has he been diagnosed with cancer or TB?
- Drug history and allergies. Ask about any analgesics he may be taking.
- Take the social history. Ask about work and what impact the back pain is having on his work. Conversely, the pain may be caused by occupational strain injury. Reiter's syndrome could be one of the

differential diagnoses (*see* Case 2) and hence it would be appropriate to elicit a sexual history.

- Family history. Ask about family history of back pain.
- Make the systems enquiry. The history of sore eyes may only be elicited at this point.
- Now confirm that the information is correct and create a problem list and a possible management plan.

Discussion related to the case

The good candidate should be able to take a detailed and systematic history leading to the most likely cause of this man's backache (Table 16). This case illustrates that caution must be exercised whilst reading the GP's referral letter as it may send you down a road that proves to be a cul-de-sac.

The clinical history here is most consistent with a diagnosis of seronegative arthropathy (perhaps secondary to ankylosing spondylitis) and renal disease is a less likely prospect.

Investigations

- Blood tests:
  - FBC, leucocytosis with infection
  - U and E – to exclude evidence of renal disease
  - ESR
  - consider HLA B27.
- Plain radiography of the spine. Radiographic features of ankylosing spondylitis include bilateral symmetric sacroiliitis. Spinal involvement initially is seen as squaring of the vertebral bodies, but with time the formation of delicate marginal syndesmophytes in a gradually ascending pattern results in the classic 'bamboo spine'.

Management

When a definitive diagnosis of ankylosing spondylitis is made, a detailed explanation of the condition and its potential implications should be provided for the patient. He should be encouraged to maintain activity. Indeed, the regular exercise to maintain mobility is the mainstay of the treatment programme. Additionally, analgesia (usually NSAIDs) can help to alleviate the symptoms. In some patients, second line agents such as steroids, sulfasalazine, etanercept may be used under specialist supervision. Rarely, severe disease may require surgery, e.g. hip replacement, spinal surgery.

TABLE 16 Causes of backache

Trauma and degenerative disease	e.g. prolapsed disc.
Psychogenic and malingerers	
Inflammatory	seronegative arthropathies • ankylosing spondylitis • Reiter's syndrome • psoriatic arthropathy. discitis.
Infective	osteomyelitis. TB.
Neoplastic	primary and secondary malignancy.
Visceral	peptic ulcer disease. pancreatic disease (e.g. chronic pancreatitis).
Vascular	abdominal aortic aneurysm.
Renal disease	carcinoma, calculi.

CASE 30: ORAL ULCERATION

Candidate information

You are reviewing patients in the medical outpatient clinic. Your next patient has been referred by his general practitioner with the following letter. Please read the letter and then review the patient.

Dear Doctor,

Re: Mr Ferhat Celik

Age: 56 years

Thank you for seeing this Turkish-Cypriot who works as a chef. I am concerned that he has been complaining or oral ulceration for some months and topical treatment with mouthwashes and hydrocortisone pellets have failed to alleviate the problem. He does have a family history of Crohn's disease and I wonder whether his bowels need to be investigated. Once again many thanks for your help.

Yours sincerely

Subject/Patient's information

Name: Mr Ferhat Celik
Age: 56 years
Occupation: Chef

This gentleman came to the UK 30 years ago and has enjoyed excellent health all of his life. However, for the past few weeks he has noticed an ulcer under his tongue, which seems to have increased in size despite using a mouthwash and steroid pellets prescribed by his GP. The ulcer is painless and there is no difficulty in swallowing. There are no other constitutional symptoms. In particular he has not noticed any fever, lethargy, joint pains, weight loss or a change in bowel habit.

The only significant past medical history is of hepatitis as teenager, which was self-limiting. He does not take any medication regularly and there are no known allergies. Mr Celik dislikes going to the dentist since he had fillings done 20 years previously. He would admit that his oral hygiene is poor and on some days forgets to brush his teeth.

He is a non-smoker but is in the habit of chewing tobacco and has been doing this since he was 17 years old. In addition, he is in the habit of drinking three pints of beer each evening but has never used illicit drugs.

He lives with his wife and two daughters, is happily married and has only ever had sexual relationships with his wife. One of his daughters suffers with abdominal pain and diarrhoea and is currently being investigated for possible Crohn's disease.

Data gathering in the interview

- Greet the patient and introduce yourself.
- Invite the patient to tell you about his medical problems. Enquire when he first noticed the ulcer and whether it is painful. Is it recurrent? Has it increased in size? Has he noticed any enlarged lymph nodes? Are there any constitutional symptoms? Ask about ulceration in other parts of the body, e.g. genital ulcers.
- Past medical history. Has he ever been diagnosed with conditions such as Crohn's disease, celiac disease and Behçet's disease?
- Drug history and allergies. Drugs such as NSAIDs, nicorandil and alendronic acid are associated with oral ulceration.
- Take the social history. Alcohol and tobacco consumption are associated with an increased risk of oral cancer and hence the risk should be quantified by asking about the amount and duration of use of these drugs. Poor oral hygiene also constitutes a risk factor and it would be worth asking about this.
- Family history. Enquire about the family history of Crohn's disease. Is it a secure diagnosis?
- Make the systems enquiry.
- Now confirm that the information is correct and create a problem list and a possible management plan.

Discussion related to the case

The possible differential diagnosis for oral ulceration is shown in Table 17. A good candidate should be able to work systematically through this list and come up with the most likely diagnosis, which is perhaps an oral squamous cell carcinoma.

Crohn's disease and Behçet's disease are less likely possibilities. Behçet's disease was first described by a Turkish dermatologist Hulusi Behçet in 1937. It consists of recurrent oral aphthous ulcers, genital ulcers, and uveitis.

Approximately 90% of oral cancers are squamous cell carcinomas. South Asians (from India, Pakistan, Sri Lanka and Bangladesh) seem to be at the highest risk, presumably because of practices of chewing the betel leaf, and oral snuff and tobacco chewing. Other risk factors include alcohol consumption and poor oral hygiene.

Investigation and management

There are no specific investigations indicated here. But it is essential that a specialist with an interest in oral cancers (e.g. ENT or maxillofacial surgeon) review the patient with a view to undertaking a histological analysis of the ulcer. If this confirms malignancy, a staging CT or MRI may be organised before the surgical treatment, which is outside the realms of this present discussion.

TABLE 17 Causes of Oral Ulceration

Traumatic and idiopathic aphthous ulceration	
Infective	• bacterial (ulcerative gingivitis, syphilis), viral (*Herpes simplex*), fungal (candidiasis).
Neoplastic	• squamous cell carcinoma.
Connective tissue disease	• SLE.
Dermatological conditions	• lichen planus, pemphigus, pemphigoid, Stevens-Johnson syndrome.
Others	• Crohn's disease, Behçet's disease, Reiter's disease.

CASE 31: ANAEMIA

Candidate information

You are reviewing patients in the medical outpatient clinic. Your next patient has been referred by her general practitioner with the following letter. Please read the letter and then review the patient.

Dear Doctor,

Re: Mrs Catherine Travis

Age: 62 years

Please advise on the management of this nice lady who is known to suffer with arthritis. She has been complaining of lethargy and recent blood tests have found her to be anaemic. I wonder whether she requires investigation of her GI tract.

Yours sincerely

Subject/Patient's information

Name: Mrs Catherine Travis
Age: 62 years
Occupation: Voluntary worker

This lady has been suffering with fatigue for several months, which seems to be getting worse and over the last few weeks there has been associated shortness of breath. Her doctor ordered some blood tests, which confirmed a profound anaemia with a haemoglobin count of 8 g/dL. There is no obvious source of blood loss. She is post-menopausal and hasn't had a period for 15 years. Her bowel habit is normal and stool colour is unchanged. Moreover, her appetite is normal and she prides herself in eating a well-balanced, nutritious diet. On a typical day she would have a fried breakfast (eggs, bacon, tomatoes and baked beans), sandwich for lunch and a cooked meal in the evening.

She was diagnosed with rheumatoid arthritis 30 years ago. The condition is well controlled under the care of a rheumatologist. Currently she is taking Voltarol 50 mg tid, paracetamol 1 g qds, prednisolone 5 mg od and methotrexate 7.5 mg once weekly. She has no known allergies.

Despite her illness, Mrs Travis is very active. She is independent in all activities of daily living and even drives a car. In addition, she carries out voluntary work in a local charity shop. She doesn't smoke or drink alcohol and lives alone. She was never married and has no children and has never been abroad.

Data gathering in the interview
- Greet the patient and introduce yourself.
- Invite the patient to tell you about her symptoms. Does she suffer with fatigue, chest pain or breathlessness? Have they developed over a period of time or suddenly? Is there any evidence of obvious blood loss (e.g. melaena)? Is the dietary intake adequate? Take a brief dietary history.
- Past medical history. Is there a previous history of anaemia and has she ever had any endoscopic investigations? How long has she suffered with the rheumatoid arthritis? Has she ever been diagnosed with an enlarged spleen? Is there a history of renal failure? Are there any features of vitamin deficiency such as peripheral neuropathy?
- Drug history and allergies. Drugs may lead to anaemia by causing gastrointestinal erosions/ulceration (NSAIDs, steroids), by causing bone marrow suppression (e.g. sulfasalazine) or by causing renal failure (diuretics, NSAIDs, ACE inhibitor drugs etc).
- Take the social history. With the long-standing history of chronic renal failure, the examiners will be very interested in her abilities to perform day-to-day tasks. Does she require home help/assistance? It is worth asking about foreign travel as certain parasites (e.g. hookworms may cause anaemia).
- Family history.
- Make the systems enquiry.
- Now confirm that the information is correct and create a problem list and a possible management plan.

Discussion related to the case
There are many reasons for a patient with rheumatoid arthritis to develop anaemia (see Table 18). The candidate must consider all these possibilities and develop a strategy for further investigation and management.

Investigations and management

Tests to consider include the following.

- FBC to confirm the degree of anaemia and whether it is microcytic, normocytic or macrocytic. A pancytopenia would suggest bone marrow suppression.
- U and E. Is there renal impairment?
- Serum ferritin, B12 and folate levels.
- Peripheral blood film.
- Gastroscopy with duodenal biopsies. If normal a colonoscopy or barium enema can be considered.
- If it is a macrocytic anaemia check for antibodies to parietal cells and intrinsic factor. A Schilling test may be considered.
- A bone marrow biopsy should be considered if the above fail to reveal the cause of the anaemia.

Management very much depends upon the cause of the anaemia.

TABLE 18 Causes of anaemia in rheumatoid arthritis

- Blood loss secondary to NSAIDs.
- Anaemia of chronic disease.
- Drug induced bone marrow suppression, e.g. sulfasalazine, penicillamine, gold.
- Drug induced folate deficiency, e.g. due to sulfasalazine, methotrexate.
- Drug induced haemolysis, e.g. sulfasalazine, dapsone.
- Felty's syndrome.
- Associated pernicious anaemia.

CASE 32: SPLENOMEGALY

Candidate information

You are reviewing patients in the medical outpatient clinic. Your next patient has been referred by his general practitioner with the following letter. Please read the letter and then review the patient.

Dear Doctor,

Re: Mr Dennis Moorcroft

Age: 63 years

I want to ask you for some advice regarding this nice chap. He recently went to donate blood, but was refused and advised to come and see me with a note from the doctor at the transfusion centre. Unfortunately, he has misplaced the note and I've been unable to get hold of the doctor who wrote it.

He tells me that he feels well and a recent blood test showed a normal FBC (Hb 18.1, plat 388, WCC 6.4), UE, LFT and albumin (39). However, I remain concerned as on clinical examination today I found moderately enlarged spleen (five fingers' breadth below the left costal margin).

Many thanks for your help.

Yours sincerely

Subject/Patient's information

Name: Mr Dennis Moorcroft
Age: 63 years
Occupation: Farmer

This gentleman had been a regular blood donor for many years, but had failed to give a donation for a number of years. Recently, he had attempted to give blood but the doctor at the transfusion service had been concerned and had advised him to see his GP with a note in a sealed envelope. He had gone to see his GP the following week but unfortunately had misplaced the note. The GP had subsequently found an enlarged spleen on abdominal examination and referred him to the hospital for specialist advice.

Mr Moorcroft has been an extremely active man throughout his life and had kept very fit working on the family farm, which he runs with his brother. Over the past few months, however, he had been troubled with a mild lethargy, which he attributed to his age and continued to remain very active. Indeed, his wife had commented on a number of occasions that he looked very well with his 'ruddy complexion'. He has not noticed any abdominal pain, bruising or bleeding. He has, however, noted an increased sensation of itchiness, which is exacerbated by hot baths and showers?

The past medical history is unremarkable except for suffering a 'ministroke' six months previously and he is on aspirin for that. He also suffers with osteoarthritis, which tends to affect his knees and takes ibuprofen tablets when the pain is severe. His only other medication is glucosamine sulphate capsules, which he buys from a local herbal shop to aid his joint problems. He has no known allergies.

He has never smoked and drinks alcohol only rarely. Lives with his wife who is well. There is no significant family history. His father was killed in an accident and mother is still alive at the age of 89 years. He has never been abroad in his life.

Data gathering in the interview

- Greet the patient and introduce yourself.
- Invite the patient to tell you about his medical problems and what he understands as the reason for referral. Has he had any symptoms related to his splenomegaly (e.g. abdominal pain, early satiety)? Has he noticed any other symptoms that suggest an underlying haematological problem, e.g. bleeding, thrombosis, recurrent infections, bruising, enlarged lymph notes, pruritis?
- Past medical history. Look for conditions that may cause splenomegaly (see below).
- Drug history and allergies.
- Take the social history. Is he a smoker? In view of the splenomegaly a detailed alcohol history should be taken (but with the normal albumin, is unlikely to be the cause)
- Family history.
- Make the systems enquiry.

- Now confirm that the information is correct and create a problem list and a possible management plan.

Discussion related to the case

There are numerous causes of splenomegaly and these can readily be found in any respectable textbook of medicine. The skill is to find the likely aetiology by looking at the clues in the GP's letter and by taking a detailed history. People are usually turned away from blood donations because of anaemia. Clearly this man is not anaemic with an Hb of 18.1, but is likely to be polycythaemic. Certainly a history of pruritis and a change in complexion to a ruddier one would reinforce this possibility.

The causes of polycythaemia are shown in Table 19. Of the possible causes, perhaps the most likely, is polycythaemia rubra vera (PRV, also known as polycythaemia vera).

PRV is one of the myeloproliferative diseases, where bone marrow erythropoiesis is increased. It usually presents in middle age and patients may be asymptomatic. Clinical features include facial plethora, headaches and visual disturbances (due to hyperviscosity), thrombosis, pruritis (typically with a shower or hot bath), peptic ulcers and in 75% of patients splenomegaly.

Investigations

Investigations should include the following.
- FBC: increased HB, red cell mass and haematocrit. In some patients there may also be a leucocytosis and thrombocytosis.
- Serum B12 and uric acid are often elevated.
- Bone marrow examination shows reduced iron stores with prominent megakaryocytes.
- Abdominal ultrasound to assess splenic size and exclude renal disease.

Management

The mainstay of management is regular venesection to normalise the Hb and haematocrit. This reduces the risk of thrombosis and improves symptoms. Aspirin also reduces the risk of thrombosis. In appropriate patients and under specialist supervision, myelosuppression (e.g. with radioactive phosphorus, hydroxyurea, anagrelide may be considered). Median survival is about 15 years, but 5% of patients go on to develop acute myeloid leukaemia and up to 30% of patients develop myelofibrosis.

TABLE 19 Causes of polycythaemia

True polycythaemia	Relative polycythaemia
Primary	
• Polycythaemia rubra vera.	• Dehydration.
	• Stress.
	• Diuretic therapy.
Secondary	
• In smokers (Gaisbock's syndrome).	
• Chronic lung disease.	
• Increased erythropoietin (renal disease, haemangioblastoma, lung cancers etc).	
• High altitude.	

CASE 33: CONFUSION

Candidate information

You are reviewing patients in the medical outpatient clinic. Your next patient has been referred by his general practitioner with the following letter. Please read the letter and then review the patient.

Dear Doctor,

Re: Mr Rupert Eldridge

Age: 82 years

Please advise on the management of this elderly gentleman. I have known him for many years and he has always been a sharp-witted man with an immaculate dress sense. I was asked to see him at home by one of his children because he had been unable to wake him up. Upon my arrival he had woken up and appeared orientated but clearly not his usual self. He was reluctant to be admitted to hospital but agreed to basic investigations and a referral to your clinic. Blood tests showed a normal full blood count, urea and electrolytes, serum glucose and liver function tests. A urine dipstick demonstrated mild proteinuria but urine cultures showed no growth. Many thanks for your advice and help.

Yours sincerely

Subject/Patient's information

Name: Mr Rupert Eldridge
Age: 82 years
Occupation: Retired carpenter

This gentleman has enjoyed excellent health for most of his life but has not been his usual self over the past few weeks. On occasions he has felt very drowsy and his son had told him that on one occasion he had failed to recognise him for a period of time and he called out the doctor. Mr Eldridge has been a very active member of the local pub quiz team and has a great knowledge of trivia. But surprisingly, on the last visit to the pub his friends were dismayed to see that he didn't answer a single question correctly. There are no other symptoms except an occasional headache that he attributes to banging his head against the wardrobe some weeks previously. This happened after falling off the chair, when he had attempted to change a light bulb. He has not noticed any weakness in his limbs, any visual problems, any chest symptoms or any difficulty passing urine.

The gentleman has never been admitted to hospital. But some years previously he was diagnosed with a transient ischaemic attack and found to be an atrial fibrillation. The doctor commenced him on aspirin and warfarin, which he has taken since. There are no known allergies.

He does not smoke (gave up 45 years ago) and drinks only four units of alcohol each week during two visits to the pub. He lives alone (his wife died 10 years ago) with two sons living close by. There is no family history of note.

Data gathering in the interview
- Greet the patient and introduce yourself.
- Invite the patient to tell you about his symptoms. Does he have insight into his episode of confusion/personality change and how often has it happened? Is it progressive? Are there any obvious precipitants (change in medication, infection, alcohol)? Have there been any falls/head injuries? Are there any features of a psychiatric illness?
- Past medical history. Have there been any previous episodes of confusion or psychiatric illness?
- Drug history and allergies. Ask about any drugs that may lead to an increase risk of bleeding (antiplatelet agents, warfarin etc). Have there been any changes in medication?
- Take the social history. It is important to take a detailed alcohol history as the elderly are prone to developing alcohol abuse, which is often associated with depression, loneliness and a sense of isolation. How well is he functioning in terms of activities of daily living.
- Family history.
- Make the systems enquiry. This is a great opportunity to consider any other potential causes for this man's symptoms.
- Now confirm that the information is correct and create a problem list and a possible management plan.

Discussion related to the case

Confusion is an extremely common presentation of illness in the elderly population. Illnesses which may present this way include infections (particularly urinary tract infections), myocardial infarction, psychiatric illness and neurological conditions. This man's history (fall, sleepiness, intellectual change, personality change and fluctuating levels of consciousness) is highly suggestive of a diagnosis of a subdural haemorrhage/haematoma.

Subdural haematomas may be acute, sub-acute (within 3–7 days of an injury) or chronic (2–3 weeks after the injury). It results from a blood clot developing between the dural and arachnoid membranes. Risk is increased by advancing age, alcohol abuse and drugs increasing bleeding tendencies.

Investigations and treatment

This man should be investigated with a coagulation profile and imaging of the brain either with a CT scan or a MRI. If a subdural haematoma is confirmed, urgent referral to a neurosurgeon should be considered with a view to carrying out a craniotomy and evacuation of the haematoma. Burr holes may be an alternative in an emergency situation.

CASE 34: CLUBBING

Candidate information

You are reviewing patients in the medical outpatient clinic. Your next patient has been referred by his general practitioner with the following letter. Please read the letter and then review the patient.

Dear Doctor,

Re: Mr Luke Stannage

Age: 67 years

This gentleman has been suffering with progressive shortness of breath for some months. I have tried multiple courses of antibiotics without any benefit. Chest examination yielded basal crepitations. Unfortunately, a course of diuretics failed to improve the situation. At his last visit, our registrar noticed that he has clubbing of the nails. After discussing the case with me today we are concerned therefore that we may be missing serious pathology and would very much value your expert opinion. Thank you.

Yours sincerely

Subject/Patient's information

Name: Mr Luke Stannage
Age: 67 years
Occupation: Retired plumber

This gentleman has been suffering with shortness of breath for some months, which seems to be getting worse and now he is unable to carry out day-to-day chores without becoming breathless. He frequently has to stop to take a 'breather'. The symptoms do not deteriorate at night when he is lying flat and he has never woken up with severe breathlessness and impending doom. There is a general malaise and he has noticed some weight loss. In addition there is a dry cough but no haemoptysis. There is no noticeable ankle swelling.

Three years ago, he suffered a small heart attack, which was complicated by an irregular heartbeat. He has been taking amiodarone, warfarin, aspirin and a beta-blocker (metoprolol) since this time. He is not allergic to any medicines.

He does not smoke and drinks alcohol only occasionally. As a plumber he may have been exposed to asbestos. Lives with his wife and they have no pets.

There is no significant family history.

Data gathering in the interview

- Greet the patient and introduce yourself.
- Inform the patient that his GP is concerned about his breathing difficulties and has referred him to the clinic for further evaluation. Then ask him about his breathlessness. Did it start suddenly or gradually? Is it getting worse? Are there any obvious exacerbating or relieving factors such as posture (e.g. lying flat)? Have there been episodes of PND? Are there any accompanying symptoms such as chest pain, cough, wheeze or haemoptysis? When did he first notice the clubbing?
- Past medical history. Any past history of respiratory or cardiovascular disease? Does he suffer with any conditions associated with clubbing (see discussion below)?
- Drug history and allergies. Some drugs (e.g. amiodarone, methotrexate) cause respiratory fibrosis. Is he on any of these?
- Take the social history. Smoking is clearly important. What impact is the condition having on his lifestyle and capacity to carry out daily tasks? Does he keep pet birds? Is there a past history of exposure to asbestos?
- Family history.
- Make the systems enquiry.
- Now confirm that the information is correct and create a problem list and a possible management plan.

Discussion related to the case

The causes of finger clubbing (*see* Table 20) should be familiar to medical students all over the world. This man's symptoms are suggestive of a respiratory condition. The most likely causes are cryptogenic fibrosing alveolitis, mesothelioma and bronchial carcinoma. Further investigations need to be conducted to make the likely diagnosis, which is perhaps cryptogenic fibrosing alveolitis. Although amiodarone can cause pulmonary fibrosis, it doesn't cause finger clubbing.

Cryptogenic fibrosing alveolitis (also known as idiopathic pulmonary fibrosis) is a rare (60 cases per million UK population) condition that has a slight predilection for males and diagnosis can only be made after other causes of pulmonary fibrosis have been considered unlikely. The pathogenesis seems to involve a complex immunological and inflammatory injury leading to pulmonary fibrosis. The trigger factor is unknown. Clinical symptoms consist of progressive breathlessness associated with a dry cough and constitutional symptoms such as lethargy and weight loss. Clinical examination shows finger clubbing (in the majority of patients) associated with fine end inspiratory crackles.

Investigations
Investigations should include the following.

Blood tests
These are not useful in the diagnosis of cryptogenic fibrosing alveolitis, but an ESR may be elevated and FBC may show evidence of secondary polycythaemia. A raised white cell count would point towards the possibility of an underlying infection.

Radiology
Chest X-ray and high resolution CT scanning will show features of pulmonary fibrosis such as reticulonodular shadowing. Moreover they will help to exclude other lung diseases such as a bronchial carcinoma and a mesothelioma. Ventilation-perfusion scans can be useful as cryptogenic fibrosing alveolitis will often lead to a mismatch (rendering the test useless when trying to diagnose a pulmonary embolus in this condition).

Lung function testing
Typically a restrictive ventilatory defect is found with reduced gas transfer factors.

Lung biopsy
A transbronchial biopsy has little value in the diagnosis but a surgical biopsy (mini thoracotomy or video assisted thoracotomy) will provide useful information. Histology shows a heterogeneous pattern of interstitial pneumonia and fibrosis.

Management

Management of cryptogenic fibrosing alveolitis is unsatisfactory and the condition carries a poor prognosis with a median survival of 3–4 years. Immunosuppression with various agents (corticosteroids, azathioprine etc) is often used to slow progress to fibrosis, but there is no data to standardise optimal start and duration of immunosuppression. Single lung transplants may prolong survival but again this has not been confirmed with research data.

TABLE 20 Causes of clubbing

Respiratory	• Bronchial carcinoma.
	• Cryptogenic fibrosing alveolitis (idiopathic pulmonary fibrosis).
	• Mesothelioma.
	• Chronic suppurative disease of the lung (CF, emphysema, bronchiectasis, abscess).
Cardiac	• Subacute bacterial endocarditis.
	• Atrial myxoma.
Gastrointestinal	• Inflammatory bowel disease.
	• Liver cirrhosis.
	• GI lymphoma.
	• Celiac disease.
Others	• Familial.

CASE 35: CONSTIPATION

Candidate information

You are reviewing patients in the medical outpatient clinic. Your next patient has been referred by her general practitioner with the following letter. Please read the letter and then review the patient.

Dear Doctor,

Re: Mrs Katherine Weir

Age: 69 years

I would appreciate your advice on this lady who has been suffering with constipation for some time. I have treated her with Sennakot tablets and lactulose solution with only limited success. She has also been complaining of lethargy and I wonder whether she requires further investigation of her bowels. I previously organised a plain abdominal film which has confirmed constipation and blood tests are as follows: urea 9.8, creatinine 146, haemoglobin 10.6, white cell count 4.9, calcium 2.8, albumin 31.

Many thanks for your help.

Yours sincerely

Subject/Patient's information

Name: Mrs Katherine Weir
Age: 69 years
Occupation: Retired cleaner

This lady has been suffering with constipation (opening her bowels every 3–4 days) for several months and has been to see her GP on a number of occasions. He has prescribed some laxatives, which have proved to be of only limited help. In addition to the constipation she has also noted abdominal and back pains and has been taking regular paracetamol tablets to try to control symptoms. Now she also feels weak and lethargic and the symptoms are causing her to become very depressed which is unusual. She has always had a cheerful constitution and never previously suffered with constipation, having a very regular bowel habit.

Significant past medical history includes a previous diagnosis of breast cancer and a mastectomy 10 years ago. She also received radiotherapy at the time and was declared disease free five years ago and discharged from follow up. She is known to suffer with diabetes mellitus, which is diet controlled and takes no medications.

She smokes 10 cigarettes a day (started smoking in her twenties) and does not drink alcohol. Lives with her husband of many years and they have a pet dog. There is no significant family history.

Data gathering in the interview

- Greet the patient and introduce yourself.
- Ask the patient about her change in bowel habit. When did she first notice the problem and is it progressive? Has she suffered with a similar problem in the past? On average, what is the frequency of her bowel motions? Is there a noticeable change in the colour and consistency of the stools? Are there any obvious exacerbating or relieving factors? Are there any other features suggestive of malignancy (rectal bleeding, weight loss, abdominal mass, anaemia)? Has there been any change in the diet and does she feel that she takes adequate fibre and fluids in her diet? Ask about symptoms related to hypercalcaemia (see below).
- Past medical history. Any past history of gastrointestinal conditions that may predispose to malignancy (e.g. celiac disease, inflammatory bowel disease)? Does she suffer with any conditions that may cause constipation (e.g. hypothyroidism) or predispose to constipation (see below)?
- Drug history and allergies. Many drugs (such as opiates, anti-cholinergics and iron) can lead to constipation and should be actively sought in the history. Also consider drugs that may cause hypercalcaemia (see below).
- Take the social history.
- Family history. Is there a family history of bowel cancer?
- Make the systems enquiry.
- Now confirm that the information is correct and create a problem list and a possible management plan.

Discussion related to the case

It is conceivable that this lady's change in bowel habit is related to the hypercalcaemia. It is perhaps more likely that the hypercalcaemia is a manifestation of the underlying pathology responsible for causing the change in bowel habit, i.e. disseminated malignancy (*see* Table 21). Bear in mind that in over 90% of patients, hypercalcaemia is due to either primary hyperthyroidism of malignancy.

Chronic hypercalcaemia leads to clinical symptoms best remembered by the phrase, '**stones, bones, abdominal moans and psychic groans**':

- **stones** – renal stones may cause colic
- **bones** – bone pain
- **abdominal moans** – anorexia, weight loss, abdominal pain, constipation, pancreatitis, peptic ulceration
- **psychic groans** – depression, confusion and eventually coma.

Investigations

Investigations on this lady should include the following.

- Serum parathyroid hormone level. If this is suppressed malignancy is the most likely cause for the raised serum calcium. If it is normal or raised, primary or tertiary hyperthyroidism should be considered.
- Investigation of the bowel to look for evidence of malignancy. This may be barium enema, colonoscopy or other such as virtual colonoscopy, CT colonogram.

Management

Management will very much depend upon the underlying condition. But in the acute setting the hypercalcaemia should be treated with IV hydration, which helps to clear the calcium by filtration and excretion through the kidneys. Loop diuretics (e.g. furosemide) inhibit calcium re-absorption in the distal tubules. Bisphosphonates (e.g. pamidronate) inhibit osteoclast activity and bone resorption and are particularly useful in hypercalcaemia associated with malignancy. Other agents that are occasionally used include calcitonin and steroids.

TABLE 21 Causes of hypercalcaemia

- Hyperparathyroidism (primary or tertiary).
- Malignancy (including multiple myeloma).
- Hyperthyroidism.
- Increased calcium or vitamin D intake.
- Granulomatous disease: sarcoidosis, TB.
- Endocrine disorders: hyperthyroidism, acromegaly, adrenal insufficiency, phaeochromocytoma.
- Drugs, e.g. thiazide diuretics, lithium, calcium antacids (milk alkali syndrome).
- Others: immobilisation (with high bone turnover, e.g. Paget's disease), familial hypocalciuric hypercalcaemia.

CASE 36: FITS

Candidate information

You are reviewing patients in the medical outpatient clinic. Your next patient has been referred by his general practitioner with the following letter. Please read the letter and then review the patient.

Dear Doctor,

Re: Mr Robin Blackshaw

Age: 46 years

Please review this chap who has had seizures on two separate occasions. I am worried that he is developing epilepsy. Unfortunately he works as a bus driver and I've had to tell him to stop this until further notice and a review by yourself. Many thanks in anticipation of your help.

Yours sincerely

Subject/Patient's information

Name: Mr Robin Blackshaw
Age: 46 years
Occupation: Bus driver

This man sought help from his GP after an episode where he was witnessed to have a fit at the bus station where he works. Apparently he collapsed and had a short lived generalised seizure. He subsequently recovered and refused to be sent to hospital but was given the day off work and made the appointment to see his GP. Two weeks previously he had a similar episode while at home by himself, which was not witnessed. On each occasion there had been no urinary incontinence or tongue biting. Also, prior to the fits, he had been feeling anxious, sweaty as well as agitated and could feel his heart racing.

He occasionally gets headaches, which can be present on waking in the morning. But they usually settle down with an alcoholic drink. He has been drinking excessively for the past six months and on average finds that he gets through a litre of vodka each day. He started drinking heavily after the breakdown of his marriage, although he has always enjoyed a drink. It is now getting out of control and he realises that he probably needs help and is ashamed to admit that he drinks during the course of the day even though he works as a bus driver and risks the lives of others and risks criminal prosecution. In the past he has found it difficult to accept that his drinking was out of control and got annoyed if anyone asked about it. The GP had not questioned him about the drinking but if the doctor asks him directly, he will be honest about his alcohol consumption.

He does not abuse illicit substances, although has tried cannabis many years ago. His past medical history is unremarkable except for hypertension, which is being treated with a thiazide diuretic. He smokes 10 cigarettes per day and now lives alone. His mother died many years ago of disseminated cancer and his father and two siblings are alive.

Data gathering in the interview

- Greet the patient and introduce yourself.
- Tell the patient that his GP has referred him following a seizure and ask him to provide you with more details about this. Terminology is extremely important and terms such as fit, faint, syncope, collapse, 'shakes' and seizure can mean different things to a health professional and a patient. It is very important to be categorical about what a patient means when a certain descriptive term is used. What exactly happened during the seizure? Were there any extenuating circumstances before the event such as excess fatigue, sleeplessness, mood changes, illness, drug use? Were there any prodromal symptoms (e.g. aura) before the seizure? Does he have any memory of the event or did he black out completely? During the event, was there any tongue biting, loss of bladder or bowel control and was there any resultant injury? Were there any symptoms following the seizure such as lethargy, headache, confusion, abnormal speech, focal weakness (Todd's paralysis)?
- Past medical history. Ask about any history of meningitis, encephalitis, head injury or cerebrovascular disease. Hypoglycaemic episodes and arrhythmias may result in collapses that mimic seizures. Is there a past history of these conditions? Does he have a history of alcohol or drug abuse? If the answer is yes, take a detailed history of abuse.

- Drug history and allergies.
- Take the social history. Alcohol history and use of recreational drugs is very important and a detailed history has to be taken.
- Family history.
- Make the systems enquiry.
- Now confirm that the information is correct and create a problem list and a possible management plan.

Discussion related to the case

Epilepsy is a possible diagnosis. But the history of alcohol abuse makes the more likely diagnosis to be alcohol withdrawal syndrome. Eliciting a detailed history from an alcoholic has previously been discussed in Case 25.

Alcohol depresses the central nervous system. In chronic alcoholics, these neural mechanisms are up-regulated to counteract this effect. When the alcoholic ceases drinking, these adaptive measures are left unopposed, leading to a state of hyper-excitability. Patients notice symptoms such as tremor, sweating, palpitations, tachycardia, and panic attacks. At the extreme end of the spectrum the patient can become delirious (known as delirium tremens) and in some patients result in generalised seizures. The seizures usually start 12–24 hours after stopping alcohol and only rarely go on to become status epilepticus.

Adult onset epilepsy is a relatively rare condition (approximately 50 per 100 000) and often equates to underlying pathology such as space occupying lesion, infection, and cerebrovascular disease or following trauma.

Investigations for this gentleman should include liver function tests as well as serum albumin and blood clotting to assess liver synthetic function. Other 'routine' biochemical and haematological tests are usually done but are generally normal. A CT scan of the head and electroencephalography (EEG) will help to exclude organic pathology and epileptiform activity.

If alcohol withdrawal syndrome is the most likely diagnosis following clinical assessment and investigations, then management should be tailored accordingly. The patient should be referred to an alcohol liaison service for help and support. Often in the acute situation patients are given drugs such as benzodiazepines to replace the depressant effects of alcohol. Alcoholics have very poor dietary intakes and are often profoundly deficient in vitamins and minerals such as thiamine, folic acid and nicotinic acid. Hence patients should be given supplements. In severe cases parenteral vitamins, particularly thiamine, are given to prevent the development of Wernicke's encephalopathy. Delirium tremens constitutes a medical emergency and patients often require intravenous sedation and monitoring in an intensive care unit.

CASE 37: DIZZINESS

Candidate information

You are reviewing patients in the medical outpatient clinic. Your next patient has been referred by her general practitioner with the following letter. Please read the letter and then review the patient.

Dear Doctor,

Re: Mrs Mary Harbottle

Age: 77 years

I would appreciate your advice on this elderly lady. She has developed dizzy spells on a number of occasions and has only just managed to avoid falling and doing herself serious injury. Clinical examination is unremarkable except for a soft systolic murmur. An ECG shows normal sinus rhythm and blood tests have also proved to be normal. I am at a loss as to where to go from here and hence am turning to your good self for guidance.

Yours sincerely

Subject/Patient's information

Name: Mrs Mary Harbottle
Age: 77 years
Occupation: Retired nurse

This lady has suffered with episodes of dizziness when she stands up from a seated or a lying position. This has happened on a number of occasions and she is concerned that she may fall and harm herself. The attacks are self-limiting and once subsided she can carry on as normal. There has never been any associated chest pain, palpitations or breathlessness and she has not noticed a problem with her vision (in particular there is no sensation of the room spinning). The problem started about three weeks ago, shortly after her GP started her on beta-blocker tablets (propranolol) for panic attacks. The tablets have helped with the feeling of anxiety that she had been suffering with and she is reluctant to stop taking them.

She is known to have glaucoma and is on timolol eye drops and oral acetazolomide tablets. There are no known allergies. She is a non-smoker and never drinks alcohol. She has been a widow for several years and lives by herself. She has no children. There is no history of serious illness in the family.

Data gathering in the interview
- Greet the patient and introduce yourself.
- Ask the patient to tell you about her medical problems. If the patient uses the term dizzy, ask her to clarify exactly what she means. Is it unsteadiness, vertigo (sensation of the surroundings moving), feeling faint etc? Are the symptoms worsened by head movements? Are there any problems with her ears such as hearing loss, tinnitus, and congestion? Are there any associated symptoms such as headache, chest pain, palpitations, breathlessness etc? Any obvious exacerbating or relieving factors?
- Past medical history. Does she have a history of similar problems? Is there a past history of cerebrovascular disease?
- Drug history and allergies. Check for any drugs that may potentially cause this patient's symptoms and establish whether there is a temporal relationship between the initiation of the drug and symptom onset.
- Take the social history. It is not unusual for elderly ladies to abuse alcohol and the candidate should never have stereotypical preconceptions.
- Family history.
- Make the systems enquiry.
- Now confirm that the information is correct and create a problem list and a possible management plan.

Discussion related to the case
Dizziness is a vague term to describe a myriad of symptoms, most often related to postural instability. Arbitrarily, it may be described as acute (present for less than a month), or chronic. When eliciting the history from a patient suffering with dizziness, it is perhaps best to consider the different 'categories' of dizziness as outlined here:

Vertigo

There is a sense of spinning of either the patient (subjective vertigo) or the environment (objective vertigo). It is usually associated with nystagmus and is often related to problems with the vestibular system. Causes include the following.

- Ménière's disease: excessive build up of fluid in the inner ear.
- Inflammation of the inner ear, e.g. associated with acute vestibular neuronitis, or labyrinthitis.
- Benign paroxysmal positional vertigo (BPPV): the vertigo is associated with a change in head position.
- Acoustic neuroma.
- Vestibular migraine.

Presyncope

Feeling of faintness or light-headedness. The patient feels that they will imminently lose consciousness. Causes include the following.

- Orthostatic hypotension: there is a drop in blood pressure on rising. Elderly patients are prone to this problem.
- Cardiac arrhythmias.
- Hyperventilation and anxiety.

Disequilibrium

Loss of balance on walking. Causes include the following.

- Vestibular disease.
- Joint and muscle problems.
- Sensory disorders, e.g. loss of vision, peripheral neuropathy.
- Drugs such as sedatives and anticonvulsants.

In elderly patients, the picture can be mixed, particularly when secondary to conditions such as cervical spondylosis and vertebrobasilar insufficiency. For this reason, chronic dizziness in older patients may be considered a geriatric syndrome. However, it is likely that the patient described in the case above is suffering from orthostatic hypotension, which has been exacerbated by the beta-blocker tablets. Acetazolomide can cause dizziness but she has been taking this drug for some time and the symptoms have only started recently.

To assess the patient for orthostatic hypotension, blood pressure and heart rate measurements should be taken while the patient is lying flat and on standing up. A mean arterial blood pressure drop of greater than

20% is strongly suggestive of postural hypotension. Initial management of this patient may be the withdrawal of the beta-blockers and starting the patient on a different anxiolytic drug if necessary.

CASE 38: FACIAL PAIN

Candidate information

You are reviewing patients in the medical admissions unit. Your next patient has been referred by her general practitioner with the following letter. Please read the letter and then review the patient.

Dear Doctor,

Re: Mrs Frances Chatterjee

Age: 54 years

We would value your advice for this lady who has presented with facial pain. I wonder whether this represents giant cell arteritis and that the patient should therefore be commenced on steroid tablets. Many thanks for your help.

Yours sincerely

Subject/Patient's information

Name: Mrs Frances Chatterjee
Age: 54 years
Occupation: Sales assistant

This lady works in a large department store on the cosmetics counter, but she has had to take several weeks off work with recurrent episodes of a searing facial pain. The pain comes out of the blue, is incredibly intense in nature and affects the left side of her face. It usually lasts about 30 seconds and is often followed by a dull ache. There are no obvious triggering factors, although on one occasion a gust of cold air had set it off. There are no associated visual symptoms or headache. She first experienced the pain three months ago. It had been an isolated incident. But, over the last month, she has had many attacks, and over the last few weeks, 3–4 attacks each day. The pain is making it impossible for her to function normally. Today the pain was very severe and she had decided to seek medical help.

In the past she enjoyed good health, having never been admitted to hospital. However, at the age of 35 years, she had a procedure on her cervix to remove malignant cells and last year had extensive cosmetic dental work.

She does not take any medication regularly, but is in the habit of taking evening primrose oil and cod liver oil as dietary supplements. As a teenager she suffered a severe allergic reaction to sulphonamides.

She smokes approximately five cigarettes each day and drinks a bottle of white wine over the course of the week. She lives with her husband, and her two children are at university. One of her babies was stillborn. There is no other family history of note; indeed, both parents and maternal grandmother are still alive.

Data gathering in the interview

- Greet the patient and introduce yourself.
- Ask the patient to tell you about the pain she has been experiencing. Ask her to explain the nature, site and the intensity of the pain. Are there any obvious triggering or relieving factors? When did the symptoms first start? Are there any associated symptoms such as headache or visual disturbance?
- Past medical history. Has she experienced similar problems in the past?
- Drug history and allergies. Are there any medications which alleviate the symptoms?
- Take the social history. What is the impact of this condition on the patient's quality of life and work?
- Family history.
- Make the systems enquiry.
- Now confirm that the information is correct and create a problem list and a possible management plan.

Discussion related to the case

This case illustrates that certain conditions can be diagnosed on the basis of the clinical history alone. Trigeminal neuralgia ('tic douloureux') is one such condition. It is characterised by intense paroxysms of unilateral facial pain, which can last up to two minutes. Patients can have many attacks during the course of the day, which has a profound effect on the quality of their lives. The cause is uncertain in the majority of patients. But, in some patients, it can be associated with compression of the trigeminal nerve (e.g. by tumours or aberrant blood vessels) at the cerebellopontine angle. Usually only one or sometimes two divisions of the nerve are affected, leading to symptoms in the respective dermatomes. Certain actions such as talking, chewing, touching face or cold air on the face can trigger an attack.

Investigations and management

As suggested above, investigations for this condition are usually not necessary and patients can be treated on the basis of the clinical history alone. Some physicians, however, may choose to investigate the patient (e.g. with MRI scanning) to explore the possibility of nerve compression.

Management for trigeminal neuralgia has been revolutionised with carbamazepine. This reduces or abolishes symptoms in the majority of patients. Phenytoin and benzodiazepines have also been used, but less successfully. In patients with severe symptoms, not responding to pharmacotherapy, more radical measures such as ganglion blockade may be considered. An alternative is percutaneous radiofrequency ablation of a portion of the trigeminal ganglion by an experienced neurosurgeon.

CASE 39: HIRSUITISM

Candidate information

You are reviewing patients in the medical outpatient clinic. Your next patient has been referred by her general practitioner with the following letter. Please read the letter and then review the patient.

Dear Doctor,

Re: Miss Sameena Dad

Age: 18 years

I would value your opinion regarding this young lady who is complaining of hirsuitism which she finds unsightly and is employing methods to camouflage. I wonder whether there is a hormonal problem that requires investigation. Her only significant past medical history is of epilepsy, which is well controlled on medication. Clinical examination, including her blood pressure, was unremarkable. Once again thank you for your help.

Yours sincerely

Subject/Patient's information

Name: Miss Sameena Dad
Age: 18 years
Occupation: Student

This young lady has sought medical advice from her GP regarding hirsuitism. She first noticed excessive body and facial hair in her mid-teens and the problem has progressively worsened since then. She has hair on her abdomen and around her nipples. But because she dresses conservatively and has never had an intimate relationship this has never posed a problem. Of greater concern is the facial hair in a beard distribution. She was frequently teased and bullied at school and since then manually removes the hair on her chin and bleaches those on the side of her face. She also struggles with her weight and remains slightly overweight despite aggressive dieting and frequent exercise.

Miss Dad had her first period at the age of 11 years. Periods tend to be very irregular and generally light, only lasting 2–3 days. Three years ago, she suffered with several partial seizures which affected her left arm and was commenced on carbamazepine, which she is still taking. She has no known allergies and there is no other medical history of note. She does not drink alcohol or smoke cigarettes. She lives with her parents who are well.

Data gathering in the interview
- Greet the patient and introduce yourself.
- Explain to the patient that her GP has referred her because of her concerns related to excess hair. Invite her to tell you more about her concerns. When did she first notice the excess hair? What parts of the body are affected? How does she treat the problem? Has she had any menstrual irregularities? Has she noticed any change in her genitals (This is an indirect way to ask if she has noticed cliteromegaly)?
- Past medical history. Does she suffer with any of the conditions known to cause hirsuitism (see discussion below)?
- Drug history and allergies. Is she taking any medicines known to causes hirsuitism (see discussion below)?
- Take the social history. What is the impact of this condition on the patient's quality of life and work?
- Family history. It is very important to enquire whether other female members of the family complain of excessive body and facial hair.
- Make the systems enquiry.
- Now confirm that the information is correct and create a problem list and a possible management plan.

Discussion related to the case
Hirsuitism can be defined as excessive male pattern hair growth in women. **Hypertrichosis**, on the other hand, refers to excessive hair growth that may occur in either men or women. **Virilism** refers to the development of male secondary sexual characteristics in addition to hirsuitism in women. The causes of hirsuitism are well recognised and are shown in Table 22.

A good candidate should be able to systematically work through this list to identify the most like causes for this lady's hirsuitism. In certain populations, such as some women of Mediterranean or Middle Eastern (including the Indian Subcontinent) origin, familial hirsuitism is both typical and natural and hence it is very important to enquire whether other members of the family suffer similar problems.

Although phenytoin is associated with hirsuites, carbamazepine is not. Indeed it is more likely to cause alopecia. In any case the symptoms started before she started taking the drug.

Androgen producing tumours would cause the hirsuitism to develop over a short time. This isn't the case here. The hirsuitism is long standing and coupled with the fact that there is a problem with obesity and menstrual irregularities, the most likely cause of the problem is polycystic ovarian syndrome (PCOS, Stein-Leventhal syndrome). Although Cushing's syndrome and late onset CAH are possible, they are but much less likely alternatives.

PCOS occurs among all races and affects up to 10% of women, making it the most common cause of hirsuitism in women, as well as a leading cause of infertility. In this condition the ovaries are stimulated to produce an excessive amount of androgens (particularly testosterone). This is secondary to either hyperinsulinaemia (leading to increased GnRH pulse frequency) or through the excessive release of luteinising hormone by the pituitary gland. The net result is the hyperplasia of ovarian thecal cells leading to multiple follicular cysts associated with anovulation.

Investigations

Investigations should include ovarian ultrasonography, which would be expected to confirm multiple 3–5 mm ovarian cysts. Hormonal studies, such as the following, also need to be undertaken.

- Serum testosterone and dehydroepiandrosterone sulfate (DHEA-S) levels.
- Luteinising hormone (LH) and follicle-stimulating hormone (FSH) levels. In women with PCOS the LH/FSH ratio is typically >2. But women with late-onset CAH usually have a normal LH/FSH ratio.
- Early morning 17-hydroxyprogersterone levels can be used to screen for late onset CAH.

If Cushing's disease is suspected, the 24 hour urinary free cortisol can be tested or alternatively an overnight dexamethasone suppression test can be carried out. These patients are prone to the development of glucose intolerance and hence an oral glucose tolerance test (OGTT) should be considered. If there is a suspicion that the hirsuitism is secondary to more complex ovarian, adrenal or pituitary pathology then more detailed radiological tests such as CT and MRI need to be carried out.

Management

Management of PCOS is aimed at correcting metabolic derangement and helping with the cosmetic problems associated with obesity and hirsuitism. Infertility and menstrual irregularities are also very important considerations in these patients. Treatments to consider include the following.

- **Hirsuitism.** Various treatments can be employed to camouflage or remove hair (e.g. electrolysis and laser treatments). Non-androgenic oral contraceptive pills and spironolactone will also help to reduce the degree of hirsuitism. Oral contraceptive pills will also help to regulate menstruation.
- **Infertility.** A combination of metformin and clomiphene will restore ovulation in over 75% of women.
- **Metabolic derangement.** Dietary restrictions and regular exercise dramatically improve insulin resistance and may restore ovulation and improve hirsuitism. Metformin also helps with the metabolic derangement.

TABLE 22 Causes of hirsuitism

Physiological	• familial, racial, old age.
Drugs	• cyclosporine, minoxidil, phenytoin, testosterone, progesterone, danazol, anabolic steroids.
Pituitary	• prolactinoma, acromegaly.
Ovarian	• PCOS, androgen producing ovarian tumour.
Adrenal	• congenital adrenal hyperplasia (CAH), androgen producing adrenal tumours, Cushing's syndrome.
Others	• porphyria, idiopathic.

CASE 40: JAUNDICE

Candidate information

You are reviewing patients in the medical outpatient clinic. Your next patient has been referred by his general practitioner with the following letter. Please read the letter and then review the patient.

Dear Doctor,

Re: Mr Eric Denniston

Age: 73 years

Thank you for seeing this gentleman who came to the clinic today complaining of dark urine. On examination I noted that there was scleral icterus, and have referred him to you for assessment and further investigation. I should say that he does have a history of drinking alcohol in excess and wonder whether this may be a contributing factor. Thank you for your help.

Yours sincerely

Subject/Patient's information

Name: Mr Eric Denniston
Age: 73 years
Occupation: Retired bank manager

This gentleman woke up one morning some weeks ago and noted on passing urine that it was darker than usual. It continued to darken further over the next few days and he decided to seek medical advice. He has also noted that his stools have become pale. Over the last month he has felt generally weak and lethargic. Moreover, over this period he has gone up two notches on his belt, suggesting substantial weight loss. He is not in the habit of weighing himself and is unable to quantify the amount.

His past medical history is unremarkable except for suffering with prostatic symptoms for which he takes finasteride. Ten years ago, Mr Denniston's wife died suddenly following a severe stroke and this resulted in what he thinks of as the 'dark period' of his life. Over several months he drank very heavily (usually a 750 ml bottle of whisky a day) and was forced to take an early retirement as a bank manager. He also ran into trouble with the police following a drink drive conviction. After this he vowed to stop drinking and has been teetotal for over nine years. He occasionally smokes a cigar and now lives by himself and is totally independent in activities of daily living. There is no family history of note.

Data gathering in the interview

- Greet the patient and introduce yourself.
- Invite the patient to tell you about his medical problems. When was the jaundice first noticed and by whom? Has he noticed anorexia, weight loss, pruritis, and change in colour of stools and/or urine? Has been in contact with anyone with jaundice or been abroad?
- Past medical history. Is there a past history of biliary (including gallstones) or liver disease? Has he ever had any blood transfusions?
- Drug history and allergies. Detailed drug history is extremely important. It is also important to enquire about over-the-counter and herbal remedies.
- Take the social history. A detailed alcohol history should be taken.
- Family history.
- Make the systems enquiry.
- Now confirm that the information is correct and create a problem list and a possible management plan.

Discussion related to the case

Jaundice can be the end result of a wide variety of medical conditions (*see* Table 23). But painless jaundice in an elderly person associated with weight loss is highly suspicious of malignancy.

Investigations

Urgent investigations for this man should include the following.
- Blood tests: LFT, clotting, amylase, FBC, UE, glucose.
- Ultrasound scan of the abdomen.

Further investigations to consider include the following.

- Liver screen:
  - αFP
  - hepatitis A,B,C,E serology
  - immunoglobulins
  - ANA, AMA, SMA, LKM
  - serum ferritin and iron studies
  - α1AT
  - consider copper and caeroplasmin but very unlikely to be Wilson's disease.
- Radiology:
  - CT or MRI scan of the abdomen
  - EUS
  - ERCP if the common bile duct is dilated.

Management

Management of jaundice depends upon the underlying diagnosis. If malignancy (pancreatic, cholangiocarcinoma) is discovered, it has to be staged using radiological tests treated according to the stage of the disease.

TABLE 23 Causes of jaundice

Prehepatic	
Congenital	• Gilbert's disease, Crigler-Najjar syndrome.
Haemolysis	• This may be secondary to **congenital** (e.g. hereditary spherocytosis, G6PD deficiency, sickle cell disease, thalassaemia) or **acquired** conditions (malaria, autoimmune disease, hypersplenism, absorption of a haematoma).
Hepatocellular	
Acute causes	• viral (A, B, C, E, EBV, CMV)
	• non-viral infections (e.g. leptospirosis)
	• drugs (paracetamol, halothane)
	• autoimmune
	• toxins (e.g. carbon tetrachloride).
Chronic causes	• any condition leading to end stage liver disease (alcohol, autoimmune, viral, metabolic etc).

cont.

Cholestatic

Intrahepatic	• viral hepatitis
	• drugs
	• PBC
	• pregnancy.
Extrahepatic	• gallstones
	• biliary structuring
	• biliary infestation (e.g. schistosomiasis)
	• cholangitis
	• chronic pancreatitis
	• malignancy causing obstruction of the bile ducts
	• (cholangiocarcinoma, carcinoma of pancreatic head, malignant
	• nodes at porta hepatis etc).

CASE 41: PAINFUL JOINT AND TEMPERATURE

Candidate information

You are reviewing patients in the medical admissions unit. Your next patient has been referred by his general practitioner with the following letter. Please read the letter and then review the patient.

Dear Doctor,

Re: Mr Roger Chapman

Age: 48 years

I would very much value an urgent assessment of this overweight chap who has presented with an acute arthritis confirmed on examination. Examination also confirmed a significant pyrexia with a temperature of 38.5°C. I am worried that he is suffering with a septic arthritis and hence am referring him for an urgent opinion.

Yours sincerely

Subject/Patient's information

Name: Mr Roger Chapman
Age: 48 years
Occupation: Factory worker

This man has presented to his GP with severe pain in the great toe of his left foot. The pain started 24 hours previously and has been deteriorating over this time. Now he is not able to weight bear on the foot and is finding the pain distressing. He doesn't feel generally unwell and has not had any rigors. Paracetamol has helped a little with pain. The affected toe is bright red in appearance and very tender to touch.

In the past he has suffered a myocardial infarct and is known to have poorly controlled hypertension for which he taking a thiazide diuretic (bendrofluazide 2.5 mg once daily). Other medication includes atenolol 50 mg od, aspirin 75 mg od, ramipril 5 mg od and GTN spray on a prn basis.

He smokes 10 cigarettes a day and drinks 4–6 pints of beer each night. He works as a steel press operator. He is required to sit at the machine all day and gets very little exercise. As a consequence he is overweight and would agree that his general state of health is poor. He is divorced and lives alone.

Data gathering in the interview

- Greet the patient and introduce yourself.
- Invite the patient to tell you about his medical problems. When did he first notice the pain? Was there any trauma? Is he able to weight bear and walk? Are there any obvious exacerbating or relieving factors? Does he feel systemically unwell and has he noticed any sweats or rigors?
- Past medical history. Is there any past history of arthritis or gout? Is there a history of lymphoproliferative/myeloproliferative disease? Any history of renal disease?
- Drug history and allergies. Certain drugs can predispose attacks of gout and should be sought. Is he on allopurinol?
- Take the social history. A detailed alcohol history is important, as it constitutes a risk factor for gout.
- Family history.
- Make the systems enquiry.
- Now confirm that the information is correct and create a problem list and a possible management plan.

Discussion related to the case

Crystal induced arthropathies cause crystal deposition in the joint and lead to severe debilitating pain. Gout is the commonest of these conditions, and is due to the deposition of monosodium urate monohydrate crystals and is likely to be the cause of this man's symptoms. Risk factors include male sex (M:F ratio is 9:1), thiazide diuretics, excess alcohol, renal disease and a diet high in purines. Pseudogout is a similar but less common condition, caused by the deposition of calcium pyrophosphate. Gout, pseudogout and septic arthritis can be difficult to distinguish as they can all cause a severe monoarthritis, associated with constitutional symptoms such as lethargy and pyrexia. Gout often presents with features of a severe arthritis affecting the metatarsal-phalangeal joint of the great toe. When presenting in this manner, the condition is described as podagra.

Investigatons

Investigations of the patient should include the following.

Blood tests

FBC, UE, ESR, urate. ESR and other inflammatory markers would confirm inflammation and may serve to reassure when treating the patient, but would not help to distinguish between the types of arthritis. Hyperuricaemia may be indicative of gout but is not diagnostic.

Radiology

Plain radiographs of affected joints are indicated and may show evidence of joint destruction. A bone scan may indicate the sites affected and a specialist may wish to obtain an MRI scan of the joint to obtain further information.

Joint aspiration

The aspirate should be analysed for microbes and crystals. This is the most useful test to decide whether the arthritis is due to a septic or non-septic cause.

Management

Management of the acute attack is with potent analgesia such as NSAIDs (e.g. naproxen) or colchicine in patients that are intolerant to NSAIDs. Colchicine may cause profound diarrhoea. Under specialist supervision, and when septic arthritis has been categorically excluded, steroids may be effective.

Long-term treatment is aimed at risk reduction:

- lose weight
- cut back on alcohol
- avoid food rich in purines (oily fish, offal)
- avoid aspirin, which can elevate serum urate
- allopurinol, once the acute attack has been treated.

CASE 42: UNSTEADY ON HIS FEET

Candidate information

You are reviewing patients in the medical outpatient clinic. Your next patient has been referred by his general practitioner with the following letter. Please read the letter and then review the patient.

Dear Doctor,

Re: Mr James Trotter

Age: 59 years

I would very much appreciate your advice regarding the management of this gentleman. Over the past 12 months he has been complaining of problems with his walking and now finds himself very unsteady on his feet. On examination of his lower limbs there is clearly a degree of spasticity and bilateral weakness. I am concerned that there may well be a serious underlying neurological problem and wonder whether he warrants further investigation.

Yours sincerely

Subject/Patient's information

Name: James Trotter
Age: 59 years
Occupation: Policeman

This man has noticed an unsteadiness while walking, which is progressively worsening, and now is unable to walk without the aid of a walking stick. The weakness was originally only noticeable in the right leg but now is bilateral. There is also a noticeable weakness in his grip and now he is having difficulty in driving his car. On occasions, he has noticed a 'flickering' of the muscles of the forearms and hands and the muscle bulk seems to be reduced. He has also noticed a slight problem with his speech and his wife has commented on the change in his voice. There has never been any loss of sensation.

Mr Trotter had a cholecystectomy and an appendectomy as a child. He is also under the follow-up of a nephrologist as he was noted to have proteinuria on a routine health check at work. He does not take any medications regularly and has no known allergies.

He smokes 10 cigars and drinks 10 units of alcohol each week. Lives with his wife and has five grown up children who have all moved out.

Mr Trotter has always been dedicated to his work as a policeman and has recently been promoted to the position of chief inspector. But his illness has had a profound effect on his ability to carry out basic duties and he is worried that he will have to take an early retirement.

Data gathering in the interview

- Greet the patient and introduce yourself.
- Explain to the patient that his GP has referred him because of his difficulties in walking and invite him to tell you about his medical problems. When did he first notice his symptoms and what are they? Have the progressed and at what rate? Are there any exacerbating or relieving factors? Has he noticed any other neurological symptoms, e.g. with vision, speech, sensory loss? Is there evidence of muscle fasciculation and wasting of the muscles?
- Past medical history. Is there a past history of neurological illness?
- Drug history and allergies.
- Take the social history. What impact are the symptoms having on the patient's mobility and activities of daily living? Has there been an effect on his abilities to work as a policeman?
- Family history. There are forms of motor neurone disease that can run in families and present at a younger age.
- Make the systems enquiry.
- Now confirm that the information is correct and create a problem list and a possible management plan.

Discussion related to the case

This man's symptoms are very suggestive of a diagnosis of motor neurone disease (MND). This condition is characterised by a progressive degeneration of upper and lower motor neurones. Unlike multiple sclerosis the condition does not lead to sensory loss and does not affect the ocular movements. Generally, there is no evidence of cerebellar or extra pyramidal signs. There is no sphincter involvement and dementia is not a feature of the condition.

There are at least three patterns of disease described for MND (progressive muscular atrophy, amyotrophic lateral sclerosis, progressive bulbar palsy). However, in real life, a patient may not fall into any one category.

The diagnosis is made on clinical grounds and there is no specific test. However, investigations such as MRI of the brain may be carried out to exclude other conditions such as multiple sclerosis. CSF examination is usually normal and EMG studies confirm muscular denervation.

The prognosis for patients is depressingly poor and most patients die within 3–5 years of diagnosis. Death is often due to respiratory failure. Riluzole (an antiglutamate drug) may prolong life slightly, but has no effect on the quality of life, and most medical management is supportive, e.g. antidepressants, enteral feeding.

CASE 43: VOMITING

Candidate information

You are reviewing patients in the medical outpatient clinic. Your next patient has been referred by her general practitioner with the following letter. Please read the letter and then review the patient.

Dear Doctor,

Re: Mrs Lesley Hoofe

Age: 21 years

Thank you for seeing this young lady who has been troubled with intermittent vomiting for some months. She is a thin lady but does not seem to have lost any significant weight. She is a known diabetic and is on insulin. Blood tests carried out by us show normal renal and liver biochemistry and there was no evidence of anaemia. I wonder whether she warrants further investigations and would greatly value your advice on this matter.

Yours sincerely

Subject/Patient's information

Name: Miss Lesley Hoofe
Age: 21 years
Occupation: Nursery nurse

This young lady has been troubled with cyclical episodes of vomiting which come on without warning. She had her first attack approximately 18 months ago and since then they have come on every three to six months. The episodes last approximately 24 hours and over this period the vomiting is severe and debilitating. But after 24 hours the vomiting resolves spontaneously and she returns to normal health. During the last episode she had associated headache and mild photophobia, which concerned her and hence prompted her to seek medical advice.

She was diagnosed with diabetes at the age of eight and was started on subcutaneous insulin, which she still takes. She is not taking any other medicines and has no known allergies.

She does not smoke cigarettes or drink alcohol and has never tried any other illicit drugs. The vomiting has never been self-induced and Miss Hoofe would describe her diet as normal. She usually has a cooked breakfast in the morning, a sandwich for lunch and a cooked evening meal. Usually she has a glass of warm milk and chocolate biscuits at bedtime.

She lives with her boyfriend in rented accommodation and the only significant family history is of her maternal aunt who died aged 46 years of gastric cancer.

Data gathering in the interview
- Greet the patient and introduce yourself.
- Explain to the patient that her GP has referred her because of her vomiting and invite her to tell you about her medical problems. When did she first notice the problem? How long does an attack typically last? What does the vomit contain (e.g. altered food, 'coffee-grounds' etc)? Are there any obvious prodromal symptoms (e.g. nausea, headache) and is there a likely precipitant (e.g. foods, drugs, activity)? Has she noticed a reduction in her appetite/weight?
- Past medical history. Is there a possibility that she may be pregnant? Has she ever had any abdominal surgery? Is there a past history of diabetes mellitus, renal disease, alcohol abuse, and malignancy?
- Drug history and allergies. Hs she started taking any pills, which may be responsible for her symptoms? Are there any medicines that she finds helpful?
- Take the social history. Detailed alcohol history needs to be taken.
- Family history.
- Make the systems enquiry.
- Now confirm that the information is correct and create a problem list and a possible management plan.

Discussion related to the case
This lady's symptoms are very typical of **cyclical vomiting syndrome**. This is not an uncommon condition that was first described in 1882. It tends to affect children and young adults but may occur in older people also. The aetiology of the condition is not well understood but a

mechanism related to migraine has been postulated, and indeed patients may experience migraine like symptoms during an episode. These vomiting episodes tend to last from a few hours to several days and patients are very well between episodes. Blood, radiological and endoscopic tests all tend to be normal, but can be conducted to exclude other causes of vomiting and to ensure that she is not dehydrated. Sensible investigations would include UE, LFT, Ca, amylase, glucose, HBA1c (glycosylated haemoglobin), OGD, and abdominal USS.

Psychiatric causes (e.g. anorexia and bulimia nervosa) have to be considered in any young patient who presents with recurrent episodes of vomiting. However, this is an unlikely explanation in this patient who does not induce vomiting, has not suffered weight loss and has a normal diet.

Although the patient is a diabetic, her symptoms are not typical of a **diabetic gastroparesis**, which tends to cause post-prandial fullness and bloating.

Management

Management for cyclical vomiting syndrome is supportive. And often the ear of a sympathetic doctor will reduce frequency of attacks. Pharmacological therapy is experimental and includes antiemetics, anticonvulsants, sedatives, prokinetics and drugs used to treat migraines. Occasionally, a trigger factor such as cheese, chocolate or monosodium glutamate (MSG) may be identified and avoiding these drugs helps to prevent attacks. Reassuringly, the disease is self-limiting and symptoms resolve after around five years.

CASE 44: UNEXPLAINED WEIGHT GAIN

Candidate information

You are reviewing patients in the medical outpatient clinic. Your next patient has been referred by her general practitioner with the following letter. Please read the letter and then review the patient.

Dear Doctor,

Re: Mrs Maria Barbera

Age: 39 years

Please kindly review this nice Italian lady who is concerned about her weight gain of about a stone (approximately 6 kg) over the past year. In the first instance, one of our dieticians saw her and was able to offer little dietary advice, as she did not feel that Mrs Barbera is eating excessively. I have asked her to start regular exercise but this is difficult as she constantly feels tired and hence I am seeking your advice to ensure that we are not missing a medical cause for her symptoms. Incidentally, clinical examination confirmed obesity and her resting blood pressure was 172/91 (I will keep an eye on this).

Yours sincerely

Subject/Patient's information

Name: Maria Barbera
Age: 39 years
Occupation: Laboratory technician

This lady has always taken pride in her personal appearance and is concerned that she has put on over a stone (approximately 6 kg) in weight over the past year. She has not noticed any obvious change in her diet, which has been healthy and low in fat. However, she is finding it harder to be as active as she used to. Indeed, she really struggles to get to the top of the stairs and often finds it difficult to rise from a seated position. The extra weight has particularly accumulated around her face and abdomen and she is distressed by the unsightly stretch marks that she has developed in this area. So much so, that she does not like her husband to see her naked, which is causing marital strife. Other recent problems include irregular periods, excessive sweating and an increase in hair on her face and abdomen.

Previously she has enjoyed good health and the only medication she takes is multivitamin preparations bought over the counter. She does not smoke and drinks approximately two glasses of red wine each week and works in a university chemistry laboratory as a technician. There is no family history of note and both parents are alive and well in Italy.

Data gathering in the interview
- Greet the patient and introduce yourself.
- Ask the patient to tell you about her medical problems. When did she first notice the weight gain? Does she weigh herself regularly? Is the weight gain associated with a change in diet? What is her approximate daily calorie consumption? How much exercise does she get each day? Is there any difficulty with exercise? Are there any activities that she has difficulty with? What is the pattern of obesity? Is the obesity predominantly central or evenly distributed?
- Past medical history. Is there any past history of hypertension?
- Drug history and allergies. Is she on corticosteroid treatment?
- Take the social history. Cushing's syndrome can result from ectopic adrenocorticotropic hormone (ACTH) production, e.g. from small cell carcinoma of lung, and hence detailed smoking history should be taken. Alcohol excess can lead to pseudo Cushing's syndrome.
- Family history.
- Make the systems enquiry. The skin changes may come up at this stage if not raised earlier.
- Now confirm that the information is correct and create a problem list and a possible management plan.

Discussion related to the case
This lady has features strongly suggestive of Cushing's syndrome. These include weight gain, which particularly affects the abdomen and face ('moon face'), striae, hypertension, hirsuitism, menstrual irregularity and sweating. Other features that may be discovered include the typical 'buffalo hump', psychiatric disturbance, and insulin resistance. Causes of Cushing's syndrome include the following:

- Cushing's disease. Adrenal hyperplasia secondary to a pituitary tumour releasing an excess of ACTH.
- Exogenous corticosteroid administration. This is the commonest cause.
- Adrenal carcinoma.
- Ectopic ACTH production, e.g. due to small cell carcinoma of the lung, carcinoid syndrome.

Investigations
Investigations for this patient may include:
- UE
- simultaneous serum ACTH and cortisol levels
- 24 hour urinary free cortisol
- dexamethasone suppression test
- imaging of the pituitary and adrenal glands, e.g. with a CT scan.

Management
Management depends upon the underlying cause. For example, exogenous steroids may be withheld if being used inappropriately. Surgical treatment is appropriate for tumours of the pituitary or adrenal glands.

CASE 45: NIGHT SWEATS

Candidate information

You are reviewing patients in the medical outpatient clinic. Your next patient has been referred by his general practitioner with the following letter. Please read the letter and then review the patient.

Dear Doctor,

Re: Mr Jake Hunter

Age: 27 years

Kindly review this gentleman who is complaining of excessive sweating (particularly at night) and lethargy. Clinical examination today demonstrated pallor and tachycardia. I wonder whether I'm missing something and he needs further investigation.

Yours sincerely

Subject/Patient's information

Name: Jake Hunter
Age: 27 years
Occupation: Office clerk

This man has been suffering with severe night-time sweats. On some nights he has had to get out of the bed and change his nightclothes. He first noticed the problem four weeks previously and there has been a progressive deterioration of his symptoms since then. He also feels generally weak and has been troubled by backache over this time. He has also noted aches and pains in his joints and muscles. His friends and colleagues have commented on how thin he looks, but he is unable to quantify any weight loss.

His past medical history is unremarkable except a tonsillectomy at the age of 12 years and a dental extraction six weeks previously. He usually smokes 10 cigarettes a day and drinks 30 units of alcohol each week. On occasions he has smoked cannabis but has never injected drugs. He lives with his girlfriend of six years, who is fit and well. There is no family history of note.

Data gathering in the interview
- Greet the patient and introduce yourself.
- Ask the patient to tell you about his medical problems. How long has he had the symptoms? How severe is the sweating? Does it necessitate a change in clothes? Is he suffering with constitutional symptoms such as anorexia, malaise? Is there an identifiable source of infection (e.g. cough, urinary difficulties)?
- Past medical history (see below).
- Drug history and allergies. Check that he is not taking any medicines that may have caused his symptoms (see below).
- Take the social history. Does he have a history of intravenous drug abuse?
- Family history.
- Make the systems enquiry.
- Now confirm that the information is correct and create a problem list and a possible management plan.

Discussion related to the case
Possible causes of profuse sweating are shown in Table 24. The most likely causes for this man's symptoms are cancers and infections. The recent history of dental extraction is very suspicious of bacterial endocarditis.

Investigations and management
Important investigations for this man should include the following.
- FBC, UE, LFT, CRP, ESR, TFT.
- Multiple blood cultures.
- Urine cultures and AAFB.
- CXR.
- Vasculitis screen.
- Consider echocardiogram.
- Lymph node biopsy if enlarged nodes discovered on examination.
- Consider HIV test after appropriate counselling.

If bacterial endocarditis is confirmed, the patient should be managed with intravenous antibiotics.

TABLE 24 Causes of profuse sweating and night sweats

- **Idiopathic** hyperhidrosis.
- The **menopause**.
- **Infections:** tuberculosis, bacterial endocarditis, osteomyelitis and HIV/AIDS.
- **Cancers:** particularly lymphomas.
- **Medications:** antidepressants, paracetamol, tamoxifen, hydralazine, prednisolone, niacin, sildenafil.
- **Endocrine disorders:** anything that causes hypoglycaemia, phaeochromocytoma, carcinoid syndrome, and hyperthyroidism.
- **Rheumatological conditions:** connective tissue disorders and vasculitis.
- **Neurologic conditions:** stroke, autonomic neuropathy, syringomyelia.

CASE 46: BLACKOUT

Candidate information

You are reviewing patients in the medical admissions unit. Your next patient has been referred by her general practitioner with the following letter. Please read the letter and then review the patient.

Dear Doctor,

Re: Miss Lisa Lowe

Age: 22 years

Your advice is very much appreciated for this lady who has collapsed with loss of consciousness on a number of occasions. Her ECG and clinical examination (including blood pressure which I am treating) were all normal today. However, I am still concerned that there may be a neurological or cardiological cause for her symptoms and hence would value your opinion.

Yours sincerely

Subject/Patient's information

Name: Miss Lisa Lowe
Age: 22 years
Occupation: Trainee police officer

This lady has had three episodes of collapse associated with a brief period of loss of consciousness. During each episode (which occurred while she was upright) she noticed a mild sensation of dizziness and a feeling that everything around her had started to spin. This was followed by collapse where she lost consciousness for about one minute before becoming fully alert and orientated. She does not recall ever having any chest pains or palpitations. She never bit her tongue or suffered with episodes of urinary or faecal incontinence.

She has previously been healthy and is currently undergoing vigorous training to become a police officer. As a routine part of her training she had a medical and was found to be mildly hypertensive and her own doctor is monitoring it. She has not been prescribed any medications to treat the marginally elevated blood pressure but is taking the combined oral contraceptive pill.

She is a non-smoker and drinks alcohol only very occasionally and has never abused any drugs. She lives with her parents and has been seeing her current boyfriend for three months. The only significant family history is of a brother who suffers with learning difficulties.

Data gathering in the interview
- Greet the patient and introduce yourself.
- Ask the patient to tell you about her medical problems. If the patient uses the term dizzy, ask her to clarify exactly what she means. What happens **before** the attack? Are there any particular situations that provoke an attack? Does she know when she is about to have one? Does she feel any symptoms such as shortness of breath or palpitations? Can she prevent an attack? What happens **during** the typical attack? Is there loss of consciousness? Does she bite her tongue? Is there urinary or faecal incontinence? How long does the attack typically last? **After** the attack is she sleepy or confused? Does she remember the episode?
- Past medical history. Does she have a history of similar problems in the past? Is there a past history of cardiovascular disease, particularly arrhythmias?
- Drug history and allergies.
- Take the social history. A detailed alcohol history should be taken and check for illicit drug abuse.
- Family history. Is there any history of similar episodes in other family members?
- Make the systems enquiry.
- Now confirm that the information is correct and create a problem list and a possible management plan.

Discussion related to the case
Blackouts in young people usually occur as a result of syncope (*see* Table 25). This is usually due to a vaso-vagal episode. Vaso-vagal syncope may be provoked by strong emotion or because of standing for too long (think of the poor soldier who faints after standing for attention

for too long). Certain situations (such as cough, sneeze or micturition) may give rise to situational syncope. Unlike an epileptic seizure, syncope is not associated with incontinence or myoclonic activity and there is no prolonged confusion or drowsiness following the event.

Stokes-Adams attacks are due to transient arrhythmias. Collapse may be preceded by palpitations and the patient often recovers within seconds. Patients can develop fatal arrhythmias and hence aggressive investigation should be undertaken if there is a suspicion that the patient has suffered a Stokes-Adams attack.

Investigations

Possible investigations to consider include the following.

- FBC, UE, glucose.
- ECG – look for evidence of heart block, arrhythmia, long Q-T interval.
- EEG.
- Echocardiogram.
- Holter monitor or electrophysiological studies.
- CT head.

If the history and investigations suggest a benign cause of blackout (e.g. vaso-vagal or situational syncope), patients simply need reassurance and lifestyle advice to avoid potential triggers. If a cardiac cause is suspected, the patient should be referred to a specialist for evaluation and treatment which may include antiarrhythmic drugs, pacemaker implantation etc.

TABLE 25 Possible causes of blackouts

• Vaso-vagal syncope.
• Situational syncope.
• Transient cardiac arrhythmias – Stokes-Adams attacks.
• Epilepsy – grand mal or complex partial.
• Hypoglycaemia.
• Orthostatic hypotension.

CASE 47: HYPERPIGMENTATION

Candidate information

You are reviewing patients in the medical outpatient clinic. Your next patient has been referred by his general practitioner with the following letter. Please read the letter and then review the patient.

Dear Doctor,

Re: Mr Peter Gordon

Age: 59 years

Please advise on the management of this chap who is concerned about his tanned appearance. He tells me that he went on holiday last year to Mexico and developed a tan, which has failed to resolve. Normally he finds it quite difficult to get a tan and I'm concerned that there may be an underlying medical problem on which your opinion is appreciated.

Yours sincerely

Subject/Patient's information

Name: Mr Peter Gordon
Age: 59 years
Occupation: Librarian

This gentleman went to see his GP because he is concerned about his skin pigmentation. He usually is pale skinned and generally does not tan easily. However, one year ago he went on a three-week holiday to Mexico and came back with a deep tan. Although the tan is not of the same intensity now, it is certainly still present and Mr Gordon read in a Sunday newspaper that skin discolouration can be a sign of serious medical illness and decided to seek medical advice on the matter. He has not noticed any other symptoms and feels generally well in himself. Indeed, he cycles four miles each day to work.

In his past medical history, he had a nephrectomy at the age of 46 years for a renal cell carcinoma, but has been given the 'all clear' and discharged from follow up. He is being followed up by the cardiologists for paroxysmal atrial fibrillation. He used to take sotalol, but this was causing excessive fatigue and was changed to amiodarone two years ago. He also takes omeprazole tablets for reflux symptoms. There are no known allergies. He is a non-smoker and drinks alcohol in moderation (usually about 20 units each week). There is no family history of note and he lives with his wife and has three grown up children.

Data gathering in the interview
- Greet the patient and introduce yourself.
- Tell the patient that his GP has referred him because of his concerns related to his tan and invite him to give you more details. When did he first notice the tanned appearance? Has it changed in intensity? Has he noticed pigmentation anywhere else (specifically ask about the inside of his mouth and palmar creases)? Has he noticed any other symptoms such as malaise, weight loss, nausea and vomiting?
- Past medical history. Is there a past medical history of Addison's disease, haemochromatosis, PBC?
- Drug history and allergies. Many drugs are known to cause hyper-pigmentation (*see* Table 26 below).
- Take the social history. A detailed alcohol history should be taken and check for illicit drug abuse.
- Family history. Is there any history of similar episodes in other family members?
- Make the systems enquiry.
- Now confirm that the information is correct and create a problem list and a possible management plan.

Discussion related to the case
Medical conditions (Table 26) may cause hyperpigmentation by causing melanin deposition in the skin (e.g. in Addison's disease) or by the deposition of another substance in the skin, e.g. haemochromatosis causes iron deposition. Drugs are a well recognised cause of hyperpigmentation (*see* Table 27) and should always be sought as a causative factor. The amiodarone that the patient is taking in this case may well be the cause of the gentleman's hyperpigmentation and other investigations may not be necessary (a routine blood screen would be advisable). A change to alternative medication or simple reassurance may be that all is required.

TABLE 26 Causes of hyperpigmentation

• Racial variation.
• Addison's disease.
• Primary biliary cirrhosis.
• Chronic renal failure.
• Haemochromatosis.
• Drugs.

TABLE 27 Drugs that may cause hyperpigmentation

By inducing a phototoxic reaction	Without a phototoxic reaction
• Antibiotics: e.g. ceftazidime, fluoroquinolones, ketoconazole, sulfonamides, tetracyclines, trimethoprim.	• Amiodarone.
	• Amitriptyline.
	• Bismuth.
	• Bleomycin.
• Cardiac drugs: e.g. amiodarone, diltiazem.	• Busulfan.
• Cytotoxics: e.g. fluorouracil, methotrexate, vinblastine.	• Cyclophosphamide.
	• Daunorubicin.
• Diuretics: e.g. bendrofluazide, furosemide.	• Doxorubicin.
	• Gold and silver.
• Dyes: e.g. fluorescein, methylene blue.	• Minocycline.
	• Phenothiazines.
• NSAIDS: e.g. ibuprofen, naproxen.	• Zidovudine.
• Others: aspirin, imipramine, phenothiazines, porphyrins, psoralens, quinine, retinoids.	

CASE 48: PAINFUL SHINS

Candidate information

You are reviewing patients in the medical outpatient clinic. Your next patient has been referred by her general practitioner with the following letter. Please read the letter and then review the patient.

Dear Doctor,

Re: Mrs Julie Beckford

Age: 42 years

I am seeking your advice on this lady who has been feeling unwell for some weeks. Additionally, now she has developed red tender nodules on her shins that have the appearance of erythema nodosum. I have organised blood tests and a chest X-ray, which will be forwarded to you. Many thanks for your anticipated assistance with this patient.

Yours sincerely

Subject/Patient's information

Name: Mrs Julie Beckford
Age: 42 years
Occupation: Cake maker

This lady has been troubled by malaise, joint pains and a sore throat for some weeks. In addition, she has now developed painful red lumps over her shins and is concerned that there is something serious going on. There has been a mild cough over the past week associated with the sore throat but no sputum. There are no abdominal symptoms or a change in bowel habit, and her weight is unchanged.

She has previously had a cholecystectomy and a hysterectomy for menorrhagia. Is not on any regular medication but has been taking a paracetamol based preparation for her symptoms. There are no known allergies and she does not have any pets.

She is a non-smoker and drinks alcohol very infrequently. She lives with her husband and one daughter and runs her own business (producing cakes for special occasions) from home.

Significant family history includes a sister who suffers with Graves' disease and her mother is undergoing treatment for breast cancer.

Following the GP consultation, Mrs Beckford has had a chest X-ray. The radiographer who performed the procedure assured her that there was no obvious abnormality on the chest X-ray.

Data gathering in the interview

- Greet the patient and introduce yourself.
- Invite the patient to tell you about her medical problems. You should look to explore two separate lines of enquiry: First, questions directed to understand the nature of the skin lesions, i.e. to confirm the likelihood of this being erythema nodosum. Second, questions related to the possibility of an associated illness, which have caused her to feel ill for some weeks.
- Past medical history. Possible causes of erythema nodosum are listed in Table 28 below. You should specifically ask about TB, sarcoidosis, malignancy and inflammatory bowel disease.
- Drug history and allergies. Is she on antibiotics?
- Take the social history. Has there been any travel abroad that may have led her to pick up an exotic infection.
- Family history. Is there any history of similar episodes in other family members? Is there family history of inflammatory bowel disease?
- Make the systems enquiry.
- Now confirm that the information is correct and create a problem list and a possible management plan.

Discussion related to the case

Erythema nodosum is a classical case for both the medical finals and the MRCP exam. You should have a good working knowledge of the condition, not least because it is occasionally seen in clinical practice.

Erythema nodosum characteristically presents with tender raised, red nodules on the shins (but can occur elsewhere). It is described as a septal panniculitis: inflammation of the septae in the subcutaneous fat. There is no vasculitis and it usually resolves without atrophy or scarring. Evidence points to this being a Type IV delayed hypersensitivity reaction to a number of different antigens. Hence, a number of conditions can cause the development of erythema nodosum (*see* Table 28). However, the cause is not found in 50% of cases and it is labelled as idiopathic. The commonest recognised cause is streptococcal pharyngitis, which is likely to be responsible for the erythema nodosum eruption in the case described above.

Investigations and management

Diagnostic evaluation should include the following tests.

- FBC.
- Inflammatory markers (ESR, CRP).
- Testing for streptococcal infection (i.e. throat culture, PCR, antistreptolysin-O titer).
- CXR. To look for evidence of TB and sarcoidosis.
- If there is a suspicion of inflammatory bowel disease, a sigmoidoscopy/ colonoscopy may be considered as may stool cultures if there is a concern that it may be due to a parasitic infection.

The condition is generally self-limiting and patients usually just require reassurance and analgesia, e.g. with NSAIDs (these should be avoided in patients with inflammatory bowel disease).

TABLE 28 Causes of erythema nodosum

- Idiopathic (approximately 50%).
- Infections: streptococcal pharyngitis (up to 50%), mycoplasma, mycobacteria yersinia, histoplasmosis, chlamydia, coccidiomycosis, certain viral infections (e.g. HSV, EBV, HIV, HBV and HCV) and parasites (amoebiasis and giardiasis).
- Pregnancy.
- Sarcoidosis.
- Inflammatory bowel disease.
- Drugs, e.g. OCP, antibiotics (amoxicillin, sulphonomides).
- Malignancy, e.g. lymphoma.

CASE 49: SENSORY NEUROPATHY

Candidate information

You are reviewing patients in the medical outpatient clinic. Your next patient has been referred by his general practitioner with the following letter. Please read the letter and then review the patient.

Dear Doctor,

Re: Mr Arnold White

Age: 58 years

Please advise on the management of this chap who has been worrying me of late. He has been complaining of a non-specific illness for a few weeks with generalised aches and pains, particularly affecting his legs. Of concern is 5 kg weight loss for no apparent reason, over the same period of time. Also, over the past week he describes numbness in his toes and clinical examination confirmed a sensory neuropathy. Other abnormalities noted on clinical examination was a blood pressure of 175/99 and an odd rash on the lower limbs resembling erythema ab igne (which has only appeared in the last few weeks). Blood tests carried out recently show an ESR of 77 and urea 17.6 with a serum creatinine of 182. There is no past medical history of hypertension or renal impairment. I'm not sure how to proceed and hence value your advice.

Yours sincerely

Subject/Patient's information

Name: Mr Arnold White
Age: 58 years
Occupation: Factory worker

This gentleman has been suffering with aches and pains for several weeks and has had to take time off work, as he has been unable to lift the heavy plates used to assemble the cars that are manufactured in the factory where he works. The pain is particularly bad in his legs and he has also noted a significant weakness. In addition, there has been a 5 kg weight loss associated with anorexia and he has noticed a red rash on his thighs that seems to resemble a 'fisherman's net'.

In the past, he has suffered with malaria during a holiday in Africa, which required hospitalisation out there and is also well known to the gastroenterology team with irritable bowel syndrome. He is currently taking Colofac and amitriptyline for his IBS symptoms. There is no known allergy. He is not taking any over-the-counter medications.

He drinks alcohol only occasionally and stopped smoking cigarettes approximately 10 years ago. He lives with his long-term female partner and has no children. Both parents died of unrelated illness in old age.

Data gathering in the interview
- Greet the patient and introduce yourself.
- Invite the patient to tell you about his medical problems. When did he first notice them and are they getting worse? Has he had any similar episodes in the past? Is the weight loss associated with a reduced appetite? If so what does he eat in a typical day? Has the numbness in his feet come on suddenly or is it more progressive? Is this having an impact on his walking? Ask about the rash mentioned in the GP's letter and ensure that you obtain a detailed description.
- Past medical history. Has he previously been diagnosed with renal impairment and hypertension? Is he a diabetic?
- Drug history and allergies. Is he on any medications that may cause a peripheral sensory neuropathy?
- Take the social history. Alcohol is a well-recognised cause of peripheral sensory neuropathy and hence a detailed history should be taken.
- Family history.
- Make the systems enquiry.
- Now confirm that the information is correct and create a problem list and a possible management plan.

Discussion related to the case
This man is clearly suffering with a multi-system disorder that is affecting a number of different systems. Rapid onset hypertension, renal involvement, peripheral sensory neuropathy and a rash suspicious of livedo reticularis all suggest a diagnosis of systemic vasculitis (*see* Table 29) perhaps due to polyarteritis nodosa (PAN). Less likely causes

of this man's symptoms include: bacterial endocarditis, connective tissue disorders and malignancy.

PAN has protean manifestations caused by a necrotising vasculitis which affects small and medium sized vessels. The vasculitis causes microaneurysm formation, which may rupture leading to haemorrhage. Thrombosis may cause organ infarction. Microscopic polyangiitis (MPA) is a similar condition that also affects the small vessels. These conditions can affect many different organ systems:

- **Skin:** painful skin ulcers, gangrene and livedo reticularis.
- **Neurological:** sudden peripheral sensory neuropathy, one of the causes of a mononeuritis multiplex (*see* Table 30), CNS involvement (e.g. stroke) and psychiatric features (particularly depression) are recognised but rare.
- **Renal:** vascular nephropathy causes hypertension and renal impairment. Multiple microaneurysms and stenoses may develop in renal vessels.
- **Cardiac:** coronary arteritis may lead to infarction, pericarditis and heart failure.
- **Musculoskeletal:** non-symmetrical arthritis and severe myalgias.
- **Gastrointestinal:** severe abdominal pain may occur, anorexia, weight loss, malabsorption.

TABLE 29 Classification of vasculitis

Small vessels	• HSP, hypersensitivity reactions, cryoglobulinemia.
Small and medium vessels	• PAN, MPA, Churg-Strauss syndrome, Wegener's granulomatosis, Kawasaki disease.
Large vessels	• giant cell/temporal arteritis, Takayasu's arteritis.

Investigations and management

The diagnosis of PAN is clinical but will be aided by the following investigations.

- Blood tests. Raised CRP, ESR, WCC, normocytic anaemia, thrombocytosis, up to one third of patients may be found to have a positive hepatitis B surface antigen. ANCA may be positive.
- Angiography (e.g. renal, cardiac, mesenteric, hepatic) will demonstrate the characteristic microaneurysms.
- Biopsy (e.g. skin, muscle, sural nerve) may show characteristic features.

The prognosis of PAN is poor unless treated with immunosuppression, usually with steroids and cyclophosphamide.

TABLE 30 Causes of a mononeuritis multiplex

Common causes	Rarer causes
• Diabetes mellitus.	• Lyme disease.
• Rheumatoid arthritis.	• Wegner's granulomatosis.
• Pan.	• Sjögren's syndrome.
• Systemic lupus erythematosus.	• Cryoglobulinemia.
• Amyloidosis.	• Hypereosinophilia.
• Acquired immunodeficiency syndrome (aids).	• Temporal arteritis.
	• Scleroderma.
• Direct tumour involvement.	• Sarcoidosis.
• Paraneoplastic syndromes.	• Leprosy.
	• Acute viral hepatitis A.

CASE 50: GYNAECOMASTIA

Candidate information

You are reviewing patients in the medical outpatient clinic. Your next patient has been referred by his general practitioner with the following letter. Please read the letter and then review the patient.

Dear Doctor,

Re: Mr Tom Rumble

Age: 46 years

Thank you for seeing this gentleman who is concerned about the appearance of his chest. I have tried to reassure him on a number of occasions, but he is adamant that he is developing breasts and is fed up with the comments that he is getting at work. He has a sedentary lifestyle and as a consequence is overweight. He is on antacid tablets for heartburn symptoms and diuretics for hypertension.

Yours sincerely

Subject/Patient's information

Name: Mr Tom Rumble
Age: 46 years
Occupation: Taxi driver

This gentleman is very concerned that he is developing breasts. He first noticed the problem about four months ago and now other people including fellow taxi-drivers have made comments and jibes, which have been deeply upsetting. Both breasts are affected. There is no obvious change in the nipples and there is no noticeable discharge. He has not noticed any discrete lumps either within his breasts or his testicles (which are of normal size). There has been no loss of libido or erectile dysfunction.

Mr Rumble works as a taxi driver and tends to spend the majority of his 10 hour shift in the cab and gets very little exercise. He generally eats fast food and is a heavy smoker (up to 40 cigarettes/day for over 20 years). Each evening, he drinks four pints of beer. For some years, he has also been smoking cannabis, after being introduced to it by a 'fare'. It used to be infrequent, but over the past year he has been smoking a 'joint' every other day. As a consequence of his lifestyle, he is overweight.

His medical problems include daily symptoms of heartburn and regurgitation for which he takes lansoprazole 30 mg once daily. He has also on furosemide 40 mg once daily for hypertension and ankle swelling. There are no other medicines or significant past medical history. He is only allergic to sticking plasters. He is divorced and lives alone. His mother died of a stroke at the age of 64 years but father is still alive and well.

Data gathering in the interview

- Greet the patient and introduce yourself.
- Explain to the gentleman that his GP has referred him because of the patient's concerns related to his breasts and invite him to give you a detailed account of his symptoms and concerns. Have the breasts enlarged over a short space of time? Are the two breasts equal in size? Has he noticed any changes in the nipples (e.g. colour) and has there been a discharge? Are there any other problems such as loss of libido or impotence? Has he noticed any lumps in his breasts?
- Past medical history. Is there any recent history of testicular trauma or inflammation, e.g. orchitis associated with mumps.
- Drug history and allergies. A detailed drug history is extremely important as numerous drugs (see below) will cause gynaecomastia.
- Take the social history. Alcohol and recreational drugs such as cannabis are recognised causes of gynaecomastia.
- Family history. Familial gynaecomastia is recognised. Ancient images of the Egyptian pharaohs from the Eighth Dynasty show gynaecomastia.
- Make the systems enquiry.
- Now confirm that the information is correct and create a problem list and a possible management plan.

Discussion related to the case

Gynaecomastia is defined as any abnormal breast enlargement in males. It occurs because of increased serum oestrogen levels, or enhanced sensitivity of the breast tissue to oestrogen. It can be difficult to distinguish gynaecomastia from pseudogynaecomastia, where there is enlargement of the breasts because of adipose tissue, without any proliferation in breast tissue.

There are numerous causes of gynaecomastia, as shown in Table 31. Physiological gynaecomastia is well recognised in neonates, pubescent males and in old age and is of no significant clinical consequence. The pathological causes shown in the table are significant and it is particularly important to exclude malignancy as a potential cause. Many drugs (prescribed, over-the-counter and illicit) may be responsible for gynaecomastia and should be sought as a potential cause.

Investigations and management

Investigations are not necessary, if the patient is thought to have a physiological gynaecomastia. In others, UE, LFT, TFT and sex hormone assays should be considered. Where a malignancy is suspected radiological tests (such as mammogram and testicular ultrasound scan) may be necessary.

Management may be reassurance, cessation of the culprit drug, treating the underlying condition or therapy to reverse the gynaecomastia. Strategies, for the latter, may include antioestrogen drugs such as clomiphene or tamoxifen and occasionally surgery to reduce the size of the breasts.

TABLE 31 Causes of gynaecomastia

- **Physiological:** neonates, puberty and old age.
- **Androgen deficiency:** Klinefelter's syndrome, Kallmann's syndrome.
- **Renal disease.**
- **Liver disease.**
- **Starvation and refeeding.**
- **Hyperthyroidism.**
- **Malignancy:** breast carcinoma, oestrogen producing tumours (adrenal, testis), HCG-producing tumours (lung, testis).
- **Drugs:** oestrogens, digoxin, spironolactone, cimetidine, cyproterone, cytotoxics, phenytoin, alcohol, cannabis, diamorphine, finasteride, metronidazole, antidepressants, diazepam and others.

Useful web pages

Asthma UK	http://www.asthma.org.uk/
BMA	http://web.bma.org.uk/
BMJ	http://www.bmj.com/
British Cardiovascular Society	http://www.bcs.com/pages/default. asp
British Geriatrics Society	http://www.bgs.org.uk/
British Liver Trust	http://www.britishlivertrust.org.uk/
British National Formulary	http://www.bnf.org/bnf/
British Society of Gastroenterology	http://www.bsg.org.uk/
Department of Health	http://www.doh.gov.uk
Diabetes UK	http://www.diabetes.org.uk/
DVLA	http://www.dvla.gov.uk/
General Medical Council (GMC)	http://www.gmc-uk.org/
MRCP (UK)	http://www.mrcpuk.org/index2.html
MS Society	http://www.mssociety.org.uk/
National Association for Crohn's and Colitis (NACC)	http://www.nacc.org.uk/
National Institute for Clinical Excellence (NICE)	http://www.nice.org.uk
Pubmed	http://www.ncbi.nlm.nih.gov/entrez/ query.fcgi
The British Thoracic Society	http://www.brit-thoracic.org.uk/
The New England Journal of Medicine	http://content.nejm.org/

Index